SURVEILLANCE AND CONTROL OF DENGUE VECTORS IN THE UNITED STATES AND TERRITORIES

Surveillance and Control of Dengue Vectors in the United States and Territories

Roberto Barrera

Entomology and Ecology Team, Dengue Branch, DVBD, CDC

OpenBook
Publishers

https://www.openbookpublishers.com

©2025 Roberto Barrera

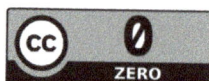

Digital material and resources associated with this volume are available at https://doi.org/10.11647/OBP.0472#resources

Information about any revised edition of this work will be provided at https://doi.org/10.11647/OBP.0472

ISBN Paperback 978-1-80511-627-1
ISBN Hardback 978-1-80511-628-8
ISBN PDF 978-1-80511-629-5
ISBN HTML 978-1-80511-631-8
ISBN EPUB 978-1-80511-630-1
DOI: 10.11647/OBP.0472

Cover photo: Lauren Bishop / US Centers for Disease Control and Prevention (CDC)
Cover design: Jeevanjot Kaur Nagpal

This book is dedicated to my dear wife and daughters, who have been a constant source of inspiration and support.
Thank you for being my guiding stars.

Contents

About the Author

Roberto Barrera, PhD, is a researcher specializing in mosquito ecology, with a focus on disease-vector ecology, control strategies, and the eco-epidemiology of diseases caused by vector-borne pathogens. He earned his bachelor's degree in Biology, majoring in Ecology, from the Central University of Venezuela, where he initiated his research on urban mosquito ecology. Dr Barrera pursued his PhD in Ecology at the Pennsylvania State University, focusing on mosquito ecology. He was a post-doctoral fellow at the University of Florida, studying biotic interactions among *Aedes* mosquitoes.

After retiring as a meritorious Professor at the Central University of Venezuela, Dr Barrera joined the Centers for Disease Control and Prevention (CDC) as the Team Lead of the Entomology and Ecology Activity at the Dengue Branch in Puerto Rico. His current work involves investigating the ecology and control of dengue vectors. Throughout his career, Dr Barrera has received numerous awards for his outstanding contributions to public health practice and programme evaluation. He has also helped various countries during epidemics and natural disasters across different world regions.

With over 120 peer-reviewed scientific articles, a book chapter, guidelines on vector surveillance and control, and extensive participation in conferences and workshops, Dr Barrera is widely recognized for his expertise in the field of ecological studies and control measures related to vector-borne pathogens.

Acknowledgements

I would like to express my gratitude to Dr Gabriela Paz-Bailey, Ann Powers, and Ryan Hemme for their meticulous revision of the manuscript. I also appreciate Mr Jose Ruiz for creating the maps illustrating the distribution of *Aedes* species, and Dr Saul Lozano for providing valuable updates on their distribution in the United States. A special thanks goes to an anonymous reviewer for their insightful suggestions. I utilized the CDC's AI large language model, GPT-4o mini, exclusively to improve the grammar and style of certain sentences. This process ensured clarity and coherence while preserving my original ideas, as well as the information drawn from cited literature references and my personal experience.

Disclaimer

The findings and conclusions in this book are the author's and do not necessarily represent the views of the Centers for Disease Control and Prevention.

List of Illustrations and Tables

Preface

Arboviral diseases caused by dengue viruses are on the rise in the Americas, with over 4.6 million cases (>2.5 thousand deaths) in 2023 and 13 million cases (>8 thousand deaths) in 2024. Infected people spread the viruses between countries, facilitated by modern air transportation. Following rises in dengue transmission elsewhere, there has been an uptick in cases among travelers returning to the United States, resulting in local outbreaks in various jurisdictions. The jurisdictions most afflicted by dengue and other arboviruses transmitted by dengue vectors, such as chikungunya and Zika, are the tropical US island territories, particularly Puerto Rico and the US Virgin Islands.

Controlling dengue vectors (*Aedes aegypti*, *Aedes albopictus*, *Aedes polynesiensis*) in the US and territories poses great challenges, because these mosquito vectors are closely associated with people and human activities. This close relationship determines the frequency of bites and risk of arbovirus transmission. However, not all mosquito species are the same. They vary in geographic distribution, micro-habitat, behaviour, ecology, and vectorial capacity—all of which are important to understand the dynamics of arbovirus transmission and vector control. This book provides a modest account of mosquito species traits, arbovirus transmission cycles, geographic location and transmission risks, methods for the surveillance and control of dengue vectors, tips about successful vector control, and key messages for dengue prevention.

The author anticipates that this book will provide valuable assistance to a broad range of individuals who are interested in the surveillance and control of dengue vectors in the US and territories. As the threat of arboviral diseases persists, there will be an increasing need to recruit additional students and professionals to address this issue. Although efforts were made to ensure that information presented on the various topics covered by this book is up to date, it is important to note that the literature in this field is extensive and continuously expanding.

1. Introduction

The most common *Aedes* (*Stegomyia*) transmitted viruses (ATVs) in the United States and unincorporated territories (American Samoa, Guam, the Northern Mariana Islands, Puerto Rico, and the US Virgin Islands) are dengue (DENV-1, DENV-2, DENV-3, DENV-4), chikungunya (CHIKV), and Zika (ZIKV) viruses. The primary *Aedes* mosquitoes responsible for the transmission of these arboviruses are *Aedes aegypti*, *Aedes albopictus*, and *Aedes polynesiensis*. Dengue was more widespread throughout the US during the eighteenth, nineteenth, and early twentieth centuries, when outbreaks were reported in Texas, Hawaii, eastern and southeastern states (Pennsylvania, South Carolina, Alabama, Georgia, Louisiana, Missouri, Mississippi, and Florida), and US territories (Puerto Rico, US Virgin Islands, American Samoa, Guam, and the Northern Mariana Islands). The geographical contraction of dengue in US states has been attributed to the increased use of screens and air conditioning, improvements in housing, access to piped water, and other public services (Schneider 2001, Reiter et al. 2003, Ramos et al. 2008, Van Kleef et al. 2010, Bouri et al. 2012, Anez and Rios 2013).

The total number of reported dengue cases in the US for the period of 2010–2024 was 55,595, of which 41,035 were locally acquired. During the first four months of 2025, there were a total of 1,568 accumulated dengue cases, with 1,389 of these being locally acquired. Jurisdictions affected were Puerto Rico (2010–2025), US Virgin Islands (2012–2017, 2019, 2024–2025), American Samoa (2016–2018), Guam (2019–2021), Hawaii (2011, 2015–2016), Texas (2013, 2018–2020, 2023, 2024), New York (2013), Arizona (2022), California (2023–2024), and Florida (2010–2016, 2018–2020, 2022–2025) (CDC 2025a). Over 90% of dengue, chikungunya, and Zika cases in the continental US were reported as having been contracted in the Latin American region (Rosenberg et al. 2018, Adams et al. 2019).

 https://doi.org/10.11647/OBP.0472.01

After the emergence of CHIKV in the Americas in 2013, outbreaks were subsequently detected in Puerto Rico, the US Virgin Islands, and American Samoa, with a few locally transmitted cases reported in Florida and Texas (Adams et al. 2019). Similarly, in 2015, Zika virus was introduced into Puerto Rico, the US Virgin Islands, and American Samoa, with limited transmission in Florida and Texas (Adams et al. 2019). The high prevalence of ATVs in US territories results from their favourable tropical climate and limited use of protective measures against *Aedes* bites, such as screens in windows and doors, air conditioning, and effective *Ae. aegypti* control. Although ATVs have been frequently transmitted in the southern US states of Florida and Texas, the lower number of cases in these jurisdictions relates to improved housing conditions (Reiter et al. 2003). In Hawaii, the lower prevalence of dengue can be explained in part by the predominance of *Ae. albopictus*, a less efficient vector (Lambrechts et al. 2010). *Aedes aegypti* is restricted in distribution to parts of Hawaii Island (Effler et al. 2005, Hayes et al. 2006, Hasty et al. 2020). It is not clear if *Ae. aegypti* was initially involved in the dengue outbreak on Hawaii Island in 2015–2016. The recent outbreaks recorded in US states and territories suggest that ATVs will continue to cause outbreaks where *Ae. aegypti* is present, and to a lesser extent where *Ae. albopictus* is present. Models predict that both species will expand their ranges further north in the US and southern Canada by 2100, increasing the risk of ATV outbreaks (Khan et al. 2020).

2. Dengue Vectors

This chapter is critical for understanding and combating dengue and other ATVs. It identifies *Ae. aegypti* (principal global vector), *Ae. albopictus*, and potentially *Ae. polynesiensis* as key vectors in the US and territories, detailing their distinct biology and behaviours. The chapter emphasizes their life cycle, habitat preferences in natural and artificial water containers, feeding and resting habits, and the resilience of their desiccation-resistant eggs.

A significant point is the influence of human activities and infrastructure on vector populations. Deficient public services and housing conditions, along with behaviours like water storage, directly contribute to mosquito production sites. This chapter also clarifies vector distribution, the ecological interactions between species (such as competition), and the challenges posed by cryptic aquatic habitats.

Furthermore, this chapter provides resources for vector identification, crucial for surveillance. Finally, it explores the complex relationship between ecological factors, climate events, and vector dynamics, highlighting the need to consider these influences for effective disease prevention. This foundational entomological knowledge is indispensable for developing targeted and sustainable strategies to control dengue vectors and mitigate the risk of ATV transmission.

2.1. Vector species

The medically significant vectors of ATVs in the US (Fig. 2.1) are the container mosquitoes *Aedes aegypti* and *Aedes albopictus*; the former species is the principal vector of dengue worldwide. *Aedes albopictus* is present in several US states, including Hawaii and the territories of Guam and the Northern Mariana Islands. *Aedes polynesiensis*, a native mosquito species to American Samoa, can transmit dengue viruses (Rosen et al. 1954), although *Ae. aegypti* is the main vector on the islands (Burkot et

  https://doi.org/10.11647/OBP.0472.02

al. 2007). Another container mosquito species, *Ae. mediovittatus*, could potentially transmit DENV in Puerto Rico and the US Virgin Islands, but it has not yet been incriminated in actual dengue outbreaks (Gubler et al. 1985).

Main dengue vectors

Aedes aegypti: Yellow fever mosquito

- Closely associated with people
- Does not depend on the presence of vegetation indoor / outdoor (resting, biting, ovipositing)
- Urban/suburban/rural areas
- Greater resistance to desiccation (eggs)
- Main dengue vector worldwide

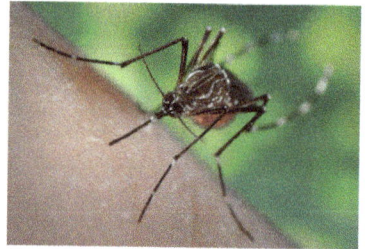

Aedes albopictus: Asian treehole mosquito

- Less dependent on people
- Depends on tall vegetation
- Outdoor mosquito
- Suburban/rural areas
- Main dengue vector in some areas / secondary vector
- Greater cold hardiness
- Better competitor in larval stage

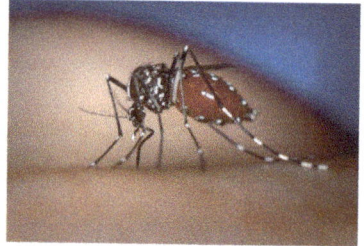

Fig. 2.1. Main dengue vectors in the United States and territories. Photos: CDC, public domain, https://phil.cdc.gov/

Aedes aegypti is a synanthropic (associated with humans), domestic mosquito that originated in Africa and has since dispersed throughout the tropical, subtropical, and temperate world by anthropogenic (human) means such as ships and airplanes. This mosquito species has both high vector competence (low threshold of infection, high rate of transmission) and vector capacity (effectiveness of virus transmission in nature) for ATVs. *Aedes albopictus* is originally from Asia and has also been dispersed throughout the tropical, subtropical, and temperate world by people (Gratz 2004). It is associated with humans, but to a lesser extent than *Ae. aegypti*. *Aedes albopictus* is adapted to a broader temperature range and can survive in temperate climates. Although this mosquito species is not as competent or capable of transmitting DENV as *Ae. aegypti* (Lambrechts et al. 2010), it is still involved in dengue transmission in some settings.

Aedes aegypti is a more efficient vector of ATVs due to its closer association with humans than any other dengue vector. This species is highly anthropophilic (prone to biting humans) and endophagic/endophilic (prone to biting and resting indoors). People in urban areas where house construction allows the free passage of mosquitoes are at greater risk for dengue transmission. All dengue vectors oviposit and undergo immature development (eggs, larvae, pupae) in natural (e.g., tree holes, bamboo internodes) and artificial (e.g., water storage vessels, discarded containers such as tires, roof gutters, etc.) water-filled containers. In many tropical urban areas, people store water or keep other containers with water indoors, such as flowerpots and wash basins, which provides *Ae. aegypti* with a suitable environment to sustain reproduction (refuge, mates, an aquatic habitat for immature development, and source of blood for eggs).

Two major contributory factors to the success of *Ae. aegypti* are: (1) deficiencies in the basic public services of urbanized areas—such as a reliable piped water supply, domestic garbage pick-up, and sewerage—that generate abundant and persistent containers with water and food for larvae; and (2) a lack of defence against the bites of adult mosquitoes in households and public buildings (e.g., screens on the windows and doors of houses, schools, hospitals, churches, markets). Human behaviour can also attract dengue vectors, for example: keeping certain ornamental plants (e.g., bromeliads) that retain water in their axils, watering plants that accumulate water in saucers, rooting plants in containers with water instead of soil, leaving animal drinking pans unattended, keeping water storage vessels such as barrels and cisterns, and exposing containers to rain (e.g., painting trays, recyclable bottles). Cavities in human constructions—such as fence poles, and uneven rooftops and floors—may also attract dengue vectors.

Aedes albopictus is a less efficient vector of DENV than *Ae. aegypti* because it is a peri-domestic, exophagic/exophilic mosquito (prefers biting and resting outdoors) and although it is highly anthropophilic, it does not rely solely on humans as sources of blood. This species instead bites dead-end hosts for dengue and other arboviruses, so its transmission to humans is limited. *Aedes albopictus* is also highly dependent on the presence of vegetation that is additionally associated with a variety of vertebrate hosts. As a result, *Ae. albopictus* can maintain populations in or around vegetated areas in suburban habitats (e.g., parks, cemeteries, tire dumps). Its dependence on vegetation excludes *Ae. albopictus* from core urban areas that are devoid of vegetation, found in many tropical, large cities where *Ae. aegypti* is the main dengue vector (Barrera 1996).

Since its invasion in the 1980s, *Aedes albopictus* has become the most common urban container mosquito in the US (Hawley 1988, Peacock et al. 1988, Black et al. 1989, Hobbs et al. 1991, McHugh 1991, Omeara et al. 1992, Omeara et al. 1995, Moore 1999, Kraemer et al. 2019, Khan et al. 2020). This mosquito species is currently found in much of the territory originally occupied by *Ae. aegypti* in the US; however, *Ae. albopictus* has extended its range further north. In urban areas where houses have screens and air conditioning, as in most of the continental US, *Ae. aegypti* has limited access to human blood, so *Ae. albopictus* is more successful because it can use alternate vertebrate hosts more efficiently. Also, lack of indoor access to aquatic habitats (e.g., water-storage containers) exposes *Ae. aegypti* larvae to competition with *Ae. albopictus* for limited resources (e.g., decaying leaf litter, micro-organisms) in outdoor containers, where *Ae. albopictus* is a superior competitor (Barrera 1996, Juliano 1998). Local species displacement has also been explained by satyrization, whereby males of *Ae. albopictus* copulate with females of *Ae. aegypti*, reducing the fecundity of the latter (Bargielowski and Lounibos 2015).

Aedes polynesiensis is distributed across the South Pacific Islands, where it transmits dengue and non-periodic bancroftian filariasis (Jachowski 1954). This mosquito readily feeds on humans outdoors, particularly in areas with overgrown vegetation that provides shelter, vertebrate hosts, and high humidity. The behaviour of *Ae. polynesiensis* is more akin to that of *Ae. albopictus* than *Ae. aegypti*. Like the other dengue vectors, this species uses natural (e.g., coconut shells, tree holes, fallen leaves) and artificial containers (e.g., buckets, tires) to undergo immature development (Jachowski 1954, Burkot et al. 2007). Other bionomics described for this species from Samoa and American Samoa resembled those of *Ae. aegypti* and *Ae. albopictus*, such as limited flight range (100m), and similarities in longevity, fecundity, diurnal activity, host preferences, and oviposition behaviour (Jachowski 1954).

Container mosquitoes are highly resilient because their populations have the capacity to recover from environmental disturbances such as prolonged droughts, freezing (*Ae. albopictus*), or vector control interventions. These mosquitoes have eggs that can survive on the walls of dry containers for months, enabling them to withstand harsh weather conditions in a quiescent or diapause state. Thus, the reduction of larvae and adult mosquitoes through vector control operations may temporarily abate their numbers, but unless the eggs are eliminated, their populations quickly recover. Another important aspect of dengue vectors is that they can exploit cryptic aquatic habitats that are challenging to locate during visual inspections, such as wells, storm drains, sumps, roof gutters, elevated water tanks, and even septic tanks (Barrera et al. 2008). Additionally, *Ae. albopictus*, *Ae. polynesiensis*, and *Ae. mediovittatus* can utilize a variety of natural containers that are difficult to locate or treat, such as elevated tree holes and leaf axils.

2.2. Identification

All three mosquito species that can transmit ATVs in the US and territories belong to the genus *Aedes*, subgenus *Stegomyia* (*Ae. aegypti*, *Ae. albopictus*, *Ae. polynesienesis*). Morphological identification of adult mosquitoes requires the use of a stereomicroscope, whereas identifying larvae requires a compound microscope. Keys to identifying the larvae of the most common container mosquitoes in the USA are available (Farajollahi and Price 2013), as well as pictorial keys to the dengue vectors of the world (Rueda 2004). There are additional identification resources on the world wide web (FMEL 2025).

2.3. Biology

Mosquitoes are insects with a complex life cycle and complete metamorphosis, with aquatic immature forms (egg, larva, pupa) and terrestrial, flying male and female adults (Fig. 2.2). After hatching from an egg, the larva starts feeding on organic particles and micro-organisms suspended in the water and submerged surfaces. Larvae go through four stages of development that require skin moulting (I to IV instars) and then become pupae, which is the last stage of development before they emerge as adult mosquitoes. Larvae can complete development in four to six days and pupae in approximately two days at 23–26 C° under optimal feeding conditions. Pupae do not feed and tend to stay by the surface of the water, keeping their two breathing trumpet siphons in contact with the air. Larvae have a gas exchange siphon and must visit the surface to breathe. Because immature mosquitoes are aquatic and look so radically different from the terrestrial, flying adult stages which can transmit viruses through biting, they cannot easily be identified as the same species, and so people often struggle to grasp messages prompting them to eliminate containers with water.

Life cycle of dengue vectors (*Aedes aegypti*)

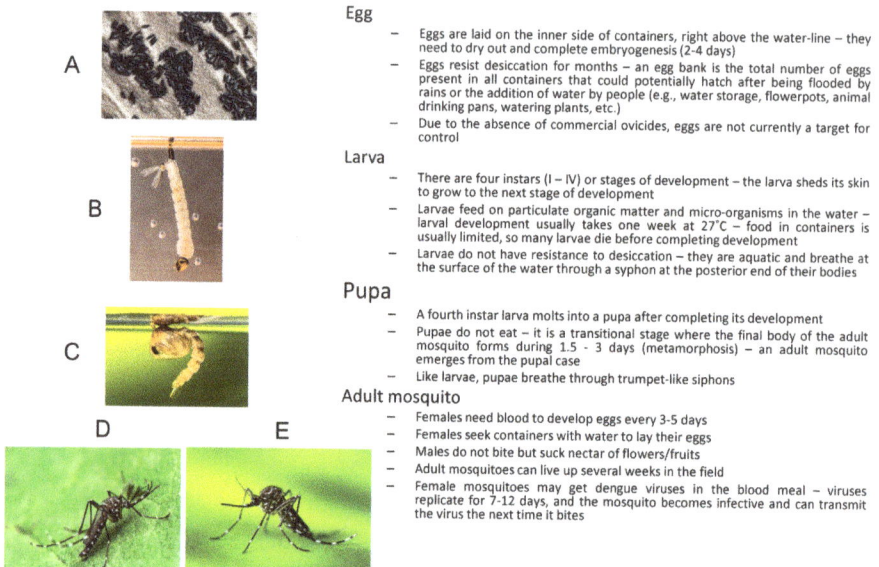

Egg
- Eggs are laid on the inner side of containers, right above the water-line – they need to dry out and complete embryogenesis (2-4 days)
- Eggs resist desiccation for months – an egg bank is the total number of eggs present in all containers that could potentially hatch after being flooded by rains or the addition of water by people (e.g., water storage, flowerpots, animal drinking pans, watering plants, etc.)
- Due to the absence of commercial ovicides, eggs are not currently a target for control

Larva
- There are four instars (I – IV) or stages of development – the larva sheds its skin to grow to the next stage of development
- Larvae feed on particulate organic matter and micro-organisms in the water – larval development usually takes one week at 27°C – food in containers is usually limited, so many larvae die before completing development
- Larvae do not have resistance to desiccation – they are aquatic and breathe at the surface of the water through a syphon at the posterior end of their bodies

Pupa
- A fourth instar larva molts into a pupa after completing its development
- Pupae do not eat – it is a transitional stage where the final body of the adult mosquito forms during 1.5 - 3 days (metamorphosis) – an adult mosquito emerges from the pupal case
- Like larvae, pupae breathe through trumpet-like siphons

Adult mosquito
- Females need blood to develop eggs every 3-5 days
- Females seek containers with water to lay their eggs
- Males do not bite but suck nectar of flowers/fruits
- Adult mosquitoes can live up several weeks in the field
- Female mosquitoes may get dengue viruses in the blood meal – viruses replicate for 7-12 days, and the mosquito becomes infective and can transmit the virus the next time it bites

Fig. 2.2. Life cycle of *Aedes aegypti* and other dengue vectors. A: eggs, B: larva, C: pupa, D: adult male, E: adult female. Photos: Lauren Bishop, CDC, public domain, https://phil.cdc.gov/

2.3.1. Eggs

The eggs of dengue vectors measure less than one millimetre in length, are oval-shaped, black, and are very difficult to see in natural or artificial containers (Fig. 2.2). Females place their eggs individually on the inner surface of vessels, just above the water line, preferably in grooves or edges where the egg remains relatively moist and protected. After two days in a humid environment, the eggs are 'conditioned' and ready to withstand desiccation for several months. Hatching occurs when eggs are flooded with water introduced by rain or human activity. Usually, only a portion of all eggs hatch at once after being submerged in the water. A lowered oxygen concentration causes high hatching rates.

2.3.2. Larvae

The biomass of adult mosquitoes is obtained during the larval period in which they feed on particles and micro-organisms suspended in the water or deposited on internal walls and on submerged objects. Larvae and pupae of mosquitoes have no resistance to desiccation, but they have some resistance to lack of food. For example, *Ae. aegypti* can withstand complete starvation in the third instar for up to twenty-eight days (Barrera and Medialdea 1996). *Aedes albopictus* can withstand starvation for longer periods than *Ae. aegypti*, which partially explains why larvae of the former species are superior competitors. In general, resistance to starvation is characteristic of mosquitoes that use small containers where food can become scarce from lack of external input, such as leaf litter (Barrera and Medialdea 1996).

2.3.3. Pupae

When the fourth instar larva reaches an adequate size and age (differentiation of tissues), it starts transforming into a pupa. This is induced by hormonal changes that determine the timing for transition. Mosquito pupae retain the ability of locomotion, but they do not feed. It is a period of drastic morphological and functional changes that use the energy stored during the larval phase to enact transformation into an adult mosquito. Sexual dimorphism can be observed in the pupal stage and includes differences in size, in that females are larger than male pupae.

2.3.4. Adults

Apart from the differences in size between males and females, there are other characteristics that allow us to determine the sex of an adult mosquito. The male has feathery antennae and palpi that are as long as the length of the proboscis. As in most mosquitoes, only females are hematophagous while males feed on the nectar of flowers and fruits. Female adult mosquitoes can feed on blood from a wide variety of vertebrates, without which most mosquito species could not develop their eggs. There are some variations in the preferred vertebrate hosts of dengue vectors, although they are all highly anthropophilic. For example, *Ae. aegypti* preferentially feeds on humans but also bites other, domestic animals (Scott et al. 1993, Barrera et al. 2012). Less domesticated vectors of dengue, such as *Ae. albopictus* and *Ae. polynesiensis*, show a reduced reliance on human blood, feeding on a variety of vertebrate hosts (Jachowski 1954, Savage et al. 1993, Niebylski et al. 1994, Richards et al. 2006). The vertebrate host preferences of dengue vectors seem to vary according to the local composition of hosts. For example, *Ae. albopictus* fed on a greater percentage of humans (76–96%) in urban areas of Rome, Italy than in rural areas (23–55%) where it fed more commonly and frequently on cattle and horses (Valerio et al. 2010).

Under optimal laboratory conditions, adult *Aedes* mosquitoes can survive for over a month. However, in their natural environment, their lifespan is typically shorter, ranging from a few days to two or three weeks (Christophers 1960, Strickman 2006, Maciel-De-Freitas et al. 2007, Hugo et al. 2010, Degallier et al. 2012). Also, males have a shorter lifespan than females. Several factors influence adult mosquito survival in the wild, including temperature, humidity, access to water and food sources (such as sugars and blood), as well as predation. Female mosquitoes require blood to produce their eggs every three to seven days, depending on temperature. While feeding on a viremic person (presence of virus in the blood), female mosquitoes ingest arboviruses that start replicating and disseminating throughout the body of the mosquito until they reach the salivary glands—a process called the extrinsic incubation period, which takes three to twenty-four days depending on temperature (Watts et al. 1987, Focks and Barrera 2007, Chan and Johansson 2012). At this point, the female mosquito is infective, and while seeking a host for a blood meal it can pass the viruses through its bite to people or other vertebrates. Because humans are the only hosts that amplify dengue and other arboviruses transmitted by container *Aedes* in the US, the mosquito's preference for and access to humans as a source of blood is a key component of the transmission cycle of dengue viruses. An important aspect of the behaviour of dengue vectors such as *Ae. aegypti* is that female mosquitoes can easily be disrupted from feeding when they detect movement or changes in illumination. If feeding is interrupted, a single infected mosquito could bite several people (e.g., kids in a classroom) to complete a full blood meal (Trpis and Hausermann 1986). All dengue vectors are diurnal biters, although *Ae. aegypti* has been observed to bite at night, particularly if there is artificial illumination (Lumsdex 1955, Barrera et al. 1996, Mutebi et al. 2022).

2.4.5. Ecology

Mosquitoes have a complex life cycle wherein immatures are aquatic whilst adults are terrestrial. For that reason, different ecological factors regulate immature and adult dengue vectors throughout their life cycle. Climatic events may influence the dynamics of dengue vectors indirectly through their impact on the quality of public services (Fig. 2.3, A1) and housing (A2). Public services influence the ecology of dengue vectors because many important containers that are used for immature development—such as discarded containers (e.g., tires), water-storage vessels (tanks, wells, cisterns, drums, jars), drains, leaking water meters, and septic tanks—depend on the type and quality of services such as domestic garbage pickup, piped water supply, and sewerage (B2) (Barrera et al. 1993, Barrera et al. 1995). Extreme weather events such as droughts may impact water supply (B1, B2) and stimulate individual water storage (B3), and in some cases this has been linked to increased transmission of DENV (Eamchan et al. 1989). A severe drought and administrative problems limiting the use of landfills were linked to a dengue epidemic in Puerto Rico (Rigau-Perez et al. 1996).

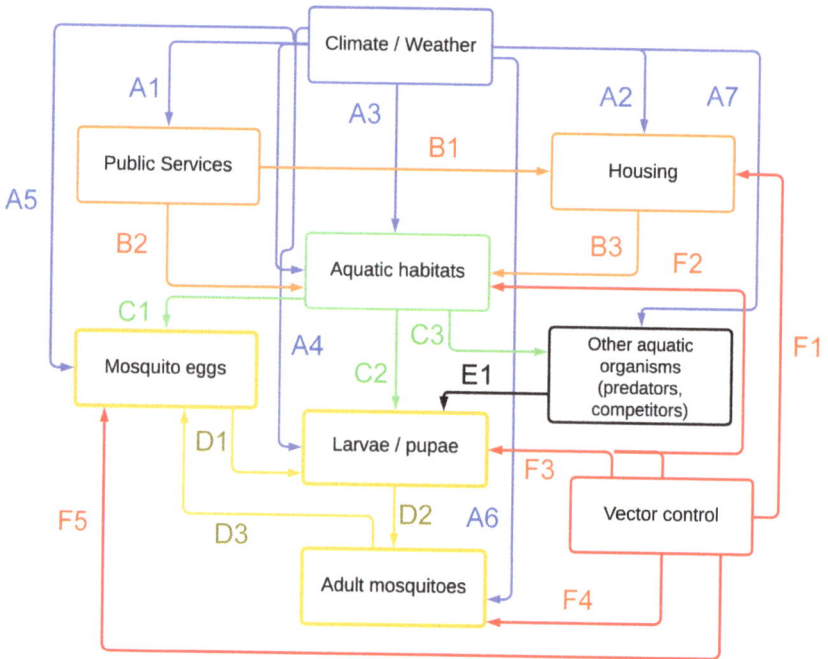

Fig. 2.3. Diagram showing dynamic aspects of the ecology of dengue vectors that explain their abundance. Path A shows the impact of climate/weather on both mosquito habitat and mosquitoes through their life cycle. Path B shows how public services influence housing conditions, leading to the availability of aquatic habitats (e.g., containers with water) for dengue vectors. Path C depicts the production of mosquitoes and presence of other aquatic organisms in aquatic container habitats. Path D relates to the life cycle of mosquitoes and mosquito population processes, such as immature development, and oviposition. Path E shows the possible influence of predators and other aquatic organisms that influence immature states of mosquitoes. Path F shows that mosquito control can be applied to mosquito habitats and mosquito eggs, larvae/pupae, and adults.

The impact of strong storms on vector-borne diseases seems to be limited, despite transient increases in mosquito populations (Barrera et al. 2019b). For example, excessive rainfall and debris from damaged buildings and urban infrastructure following Category 4 Hurricane Maria in 2017 led to significant surges in adult *Ae. aegypti* populations across various locations in Puerto Rico. However, these increases in mosquito abundance did not result in outbreaks of ATV, as the circulation of ATVs was low during that period (Barrera et al. 2019b). Previous observations on the impact of Category 3 Hurricane Georges in 1998 that occurred during the peak of dengue transmission in Puerto Rico found no effect on dengue transmission, except for brief interruptions in the reporting system (Rigau-Perez et al. 1996). The limited impact of storms on ATV transmission is not yet well understood. One possible explanation is that the subsequent number of containers producing *Aedes* is temporarily reduced in flooded areas and in general, because the cleansing of properties and disposal of debris by residents might reduce the availability of containers producing mosquitoes.

Other climatic events include El Niño Southern Oscillation (ENSO) which recurs every two to seven years, generally bringing warmer conditions and changes in rainfall in some areas (Ropelewski and Halpert 1987). For example, ENSO is associated with wetter conditions in the southeast US but drier than normal conditions in the Caribbean and northern South America. El Niño is generally followed by La Niña conditions that have opposite effects on local weather, such as cooler and wetter weather. Understanding the effects of ENSO on vector-borne diseases is complicated, but there is evidence that it influences the incidence of dengue, malaria, and Rift Walley fever (Anyamba et al. 2019). In Puerto Rico, a strong El Niño during 2014–2016 was associated with severe droughts but did not affect the local populations of *Ae. aegypti* (Barrera et al. 2023). Yet, ATV cases in that study were associated with five- to ten-month lagged values of the Oceanic El Niño index, drought extent, and *Ae. aegypti* populations. As has been observed in other countries in the Caribbean, dengue epidemics in Puerto Rico tend to occur in the year following the onset of strong El Niño conditions (Amarakoon et al. 2008, Barrera et al. 2023).

Climate has an impact on housing characteristics, which in turn influence the ecology of dengue vectors. Houses are more inaccessible to mosquitoes in temperate and subtropical areas due to the use of heating and air conditioning to regulate temperature internally, as well as the generalized use of screens. Thus, dengue vectors remain outdoors most of the time and have less access to human blood. By contrast, houses in most tropical countries favour natural ventilation (open windows, doors, eaves), which facilitates the free passage of mosquitoes, particularly *Ae. aegypti* which tends to rest and bite indoors. The use of screens on windows and doors, or any other devices blocking air circulation, are uncommon. Thus, housing characteristics and human behaviour largely determine the extent of vector-host contact and dengue transmission, as reported from a study in south Texas (Reiter et al. 2003).

The geographic distribution of dengue vectors is limited by climate and modulated by latitude, elevation, and desertic conditions. For example, the distribution of *Ae. aegypti* is limited by the January 10° C isotherm (e.g., northernmost US states), both north and south of the Equator, and by elevations above 2,200m (Christophers 1960, Lozano-Fuentes et al. 2012). A study on the distribution of ATV cases in relation to elevation in sixteen countries in the Americas showed that cases of these diseases rarely occurred above 2,000m (Watts et al. 2017). Following timely introductions, *Ae. aegypti* can establish transient populations further north in the US during the summer (Monaghan et al. 2016), which has historically led to epidemics of yellow fever and dengue (Shope 1991). *Aedes aegypti* mosquitoes are present in some desert areas where they would not normally exist, but they thrive under these conditions due to local water-storage practices (Hopp and Foley 2001). The northern limit of distribution of *Ae. albopictus* is the January 0° C isotherm or an annual mean temperature of 11° C, and transient, summer populations can extend up to the January -5 °C isotherm; but precise limits vary by continent depending on the average temperature range (Mogi et al. 2012).

Intra-annual climate variability or seasonality influences the availability of aquatic habitats (Fig. 2.3, A3) and defines the growing and reproductive seasons (Fig. 2.3, A4–7). Seasonal changes in rainfall and temperature affect the dynamics of dengue vectors and dengue (Moore et al. 1978, Johansson et al. 2009, Barrera et al. 2011). A study on the seasonality of *Ae. aegypti* in fifty US cities concluded that weather conditions during winter are unsuitable for this mosquito species, except in southern Florida and Texas (Monaghan et al. 2016). In tropical areas where people keep containers with water, the temporal dynamics of dengue vectors are more complex, with seasonal increases during the rainy season and relatively steady mosquito populations even through prolonged dry seasons (Barrera et al. 1996). Lack of natural or weather-mediated mosquito abatement resulting from human behaviour (watering plants, water-storage, animal drinking pans, septic tanks) seems to be a major contributor to dengue endemism/hyper endemism (the cocirculation of two or more dengue virus serotypes).

The quality and quantity (Fig. 2.3, C2, D2) of aquatic habitats in natural and artificial containers determine the number of adult mosquitoes at a given location and time. Dengue vectors occur at a low density due to the smaller size of their aquatic habitats that produce fewer mosquitoes than those that develop in extensive or large bodies of water on the ground. Small aquatic habitats tend to be overcrowded with larvae that compete for limited resources (Fig. 2.3, D2) (Barrera 1996). Containers typically hold an egg bank (Fig. 2.3, C1) resulting from past oviposition activity by female mosquitoes (Fig. 2.3, D3) and may survive in the containers for several months. Eggs eventually hatch (Fig. 2.3, D1) when they are flooded by rains or by the addition of water by humans.

The main mortality factors of immature dengue vectors are lack of food and desiccation. Aquatic predators (Fig. 2.3, E1) play a minor role (copepods, other immature aquatic insects such as dragonflies and *Toxorhynchites*), possibly because of the small size of containers and their short cycles of filling and desiccation. Aquatic predators require environments that are richer in preys and more temporally stable. Competition with other dengue vectors occurs in areas of overlap, as has been documented between *Ae. aegypti* and *Ae. albopictus*. Landscape and vegetation influence the composition of aquatic habitats, characteristics of the terrestrial environment of adult mosquitoes, and differential distribution of dengue vectors (Rey et al. 2006, Little et al. 2011). For example, *Ae. albopictus* is rarely found in the core of urban areas with scarce vegetation where *Ae. aegypti* becomes the main dengue vector species (Chan et al. 1971). Vector control measures, as will be discussed later, can be applied directly against mosquito eggs, larvae/pupae, and adults (Fig. 2.3, F3–5), or indirectly by improving housing and public services (e.g., reliable piped water supply) to reduce the availability of important aquatic habitats (e.g., water storage vessels; Fig. 2.3, F1–2).

3. *Aedes* Transmitted Virus (ATV) Cycles

This chapter elucidates the distinct transmission pathways of dengue, chikungunya, and Zika viruses. It differentiates between enzootic cycles, primarily occurring in the forests of Southeast Asia and West Africa, involving sylvatic *Aedes* mosquitoes and nonhuman primates. Humans can become infected through bridge vectors like *Ae. albopictus* and *Ae. furcifer* in fringe-forest or rural areas. Notably, enzootic cycles of DENV are not evident in the Americas.

The chapter then details the urban cycle, which is similar for all ATVs. In this cycle, domestic or peri-domestic *Aedes* mosquitoes transmit the viruses to humans in urban, suburban, and rural settings. Mosquitoes acquire the virus by feeding on infected persons, undergo an extrinsic incubation period, and then transmit the virus to susceptible people through their bites. The cycle can be interrupted if infected mosquitoes bite non-amplifying hosts or immune individuals. While vertical transmission in mosquitoes is possible, its role in urban endemicity is unclear. Virus spread occurs locally within neighbourhoods and through jump dispersal via infected individuals or mosquitoes to distant areas, including through international travel, complicating control efforts and promoting endemicity.

3.1. Enzootic cycles

Dengue viruses (DENV-1, DENV-2, DENV-3, DENV-4; *Flaviviridae*: *Orthoflavivirus*) circulate between sylvatic mosquitoes and nonhuman primates in the forests of Southeast Asia and West Africa (Gubler 1988, Vasilakis et al. 2011). Vertical transmission of DENV has been documented in wild dengue vectors in both continents (Gubler 1988). The main mosquito vectors involved in the enzootic cycle in Southeast Asia are

 https://doi.org/10.11647/OBP.0472.03

species of the *Aedes niveus* group, which are canopy forest mosquitoes that feed on primates (*Macaca* spp., *Presbytis* spp.), including humans. People may become infected in the forest but also in nearby inhabited, rural areas through the bite of bridge vectors such as *Ae. albopictus*, which are fringe-forest mosquitoes. Several mosquito vectors have been found infected with DENV in gallery forests in Africa, such as *Ae. africanus*, *Ae. luteocephalus*, *Ae. opok*, *Ae. taylori*, and *Ae. furcifer*. Various monkey species have been found naturally infected with DENV in West Africa (*Chlorocebus sabaeus*, *Papio papio*, *Erythrocebus patas*). The main bridge vector between forested areas and humans in rural areas is *Ae. furcifer*. Enzootic cycles of DENV do not seem to occur in the Americas. Sylvatic and urban DENV strains represent distinct genetic lineages, although both seem to cause similar symptoms in humans (Gubler 1988, Vasilakis et al. 2011).

Chikungunya virus (CHIKV; *Togaviridae*: *Alphavirus*) is originally from Africa, where it circulates in forested areas between nonhuman primates and several sylvatic *Aedes* mosquitoes, such as *Ae. africanus*, *Ae. cordellieri*, *Ae. dalzieli*, *Ae. furcifer*, *Ae. luteocephalus*, *Ae. taylori*, and *Ae. vittatus* (Jupp and McIntosh 1988, Zeller et al. 2016).

Zika virus (ZIKV; *Flaviviridae*: *Orthoflavivirus*) is originally from Africa, where it circulates between nonhuman primates and mosquitoes in forested areas, causing periodic epizootics in primates (Musso and Gubler 2016). ZIKV has been isolated from several sylvatic *Aedes* mosquitoes, mainly *Ae. africanus*, *Ae. luteocephalus, and Ae. furcifer-taylori* (Musso and Gubler 2016).

3.2. Urban cycle

The urban cycle of all ATVs is similar, wherein the viruses are transmitted to humans by domestic or peri-domestic mosquitoes in urban, suburban, and rural areas (Fig. 3.1). Dengue vectors are highly anthropophilic (Fig. 3.1, D1) but they can also bite domestic or wild, peri-domestic vertebrates (Fig. 3.1, D2). Mosquitoes acquire the virus through the blood meal taken from infected humans (Fig. 3.1, D3), becoming infective after completion of the extrinsic incubation period. Infected mosquitoes can then bite a susceptible person and transmit the virus, completing the transmission cycle (Fig. 3.1, D1). Some infected mosquitoes may bite humans that have previously been infected with the same virus (same serotype for dengue viruses) or may bite other vertebrates wherein the virus cannot replicate or survive (Fig. 3.1, D4), in which case the virus will not continue to circulate. ATVs can also be passed vertically from infected adult female mosquitoes to their progeny, but it is not clear whether this mechanism of transmission actually plays a role or how important it is to maintaining endemicity in urban areas (Adams et al. 2010). ATVs have been shown to disseminate centripetally (radiate outwards from the initial site of virus introduction) in the same neighbourhood and by jump dispersal in infected people or mosquitoes to other, distant neighbourhoods within a city (Fig. 3.1, D5) (Kan et al. 2008), or through great distances by air travel (Luce et al. 2010). The frequent introduction of ATVs to environments favourable for transmission complicates their control, because this promotes virus endemicity in new environments.

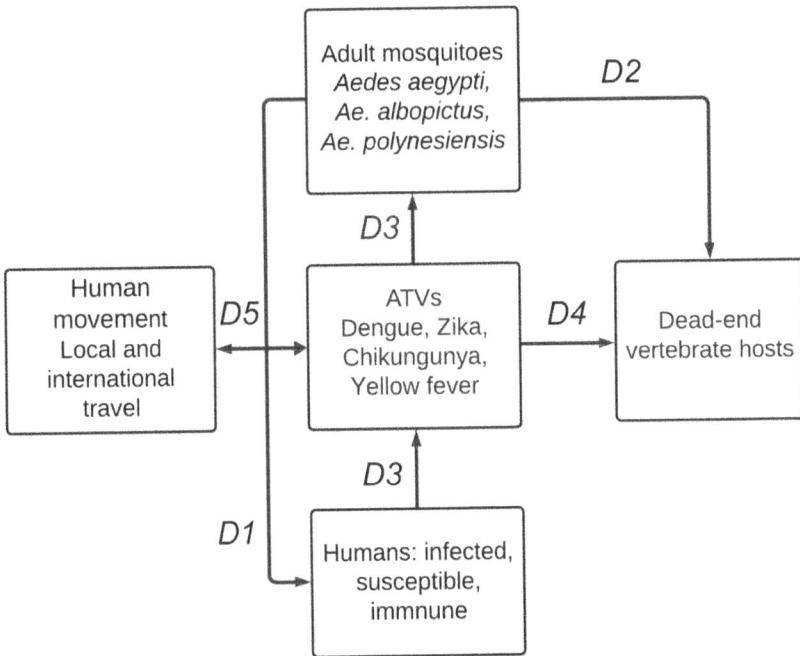

Fig. 3.1. Urban cycle of *Aedes* transmitted viruses (ATVs), showing transmission to humans by infected mosquitoes (D1). Mosquitoes feed on vertebrates other than people (D2). However, when infective bites go into vertebrates that do not amplify the viruses, or into already immune persons (D4), the transmission cycle is interrupted. Infected people infect mosquitoes during the viremic period that continues with the transmission cycle (D3). Local and international human and mosquito movements can export/import viruses (D5).

4. Risk of ATVs in the US and Territories

The risk of acquiring ATVs and the need to control virus transmission varies between geographical locations, depending on the presence and dynamics of the vector and virus populations. US states and territories are classified here with varying expected risks for ATV transmission. This classification is mainly based on historical patterns of ATV transmission, distribution of vector species, and climate. The main purpose of this classification is to allow an initial rapid assessment of the importance of detecting cases in the US.

Endemic/Epidemic areas (Puerto Rico, US Virgin Islands, American Samoa) experience ongoing dengue transmission, primarily by *Ae. aegypti*, with periodic epidemics. These tropical territories offer conducive climates and housing for persistent vector and virus populations.

Non-endemic areas with elevated risk (Southern Florida, Texas, subtropical US, California, Hawaii, Guam, Northern Mariana Islands) harbour *Ae. aegypti* or *Ae. albopictus* and have reported local ATV outbreaks, indicating potential for the emergence or re-emergence of endemicity. Frequent virus introductions by travellers exacerbates this risk. While *Ae. albopictus* is considered a less efficient vector, it has driven outbreaks in some Pacific territories and Hawaii.

Non-endemic areas with lower risk (at northern latitudes) have established *Ae. albopictus* populations and occasional *Ae. aegypti* introductions, but widespread ATV transmission is less common. Factors like housing infrastructure (screens, AC) and *Ae. albopictus'* feeding habits may limit transmission. Most cases are imported, although localized transmission during warmer months is possible.

Finally, **no-risk areas** lack established dengue vector populations (Alaska, many western and midwestern states, etc.), thus presenting minimal to no risk of local ATV transmission despite occasional vector introductions.

 https://doi.org/10.11647/OBP.0472.04

This risk assessment is crucial for guiding surveillance and control efforts across the US and territories.

4.1. Endemic/epidemic transmission via *Aedes aegypti* in the tropics (Puerto Rico, US Virgin Islands, and American Samoa)

Most documented autochthonous or locally acquired ATV cases in the US have been transmitted by *Aedes aegypti*, which is the main vector worldwide. *Aedes aegypti* is present in US territories where climate and housing conditions are conducive to persistent mosquito and virus populations in the absence of effective vector control (Fig. 4.1; Table 1). Dengue viruses are endemic, causing periodic epidemics in several US territories, while CHIKV and ZIKV have not become endemic in US territories.

Dengue transmission in Puerto Rico has a long history and can be summarized in terms of four periods: 1915–1969, with self-limited outbreaks of one virus serotype; 1969–1980, when dengue became endemic with the circulation of alternating, single serotypes; 1980–2015, with hyper-endemic, simultaneous circulation of more than one virus serotype, shortly followed by the establishment of endemic, severe dengue (e.g., haemorrhagic manifestations); and 2016–2025 when, following the ZIKV epidemic in 2016–2017, transmission was lower than in previous years (Barrera 2010; Adams et al. 2019; CDC 2025b; PAHO 2025). The largest DENV epidemic in Puerto Rico was in 2010, when there were 26,766 suspected dengue cases and 40 fatalities (Sharp et al. 2013). Dengue cases have been recorded in every month of the year in Puerto Rico, although peak transmission occurs in late boreal summer and autumn (Fig. 4.2) (Jury 2008, Johansson et al. 2009, Barrera 2010). CHIKV and ZIKV have caused epidemics in Puerto Rico, US Virgin Islands, and American Samoa, as explained earlier.

Dengue outbreaks have been documented in the US Virgin Islands since 1827, with notable outbreaks occurring in the early twentieth century, and in 1977 before dengue became endemic in the Caribbean (Brathwaite et al. 2011). DENVs have been present in the US Virgin Islands during most years (Rigau-Perez et al. 1994).

Dengue has also been frequently reported in American Samoa (Arima et al. 2013, Sharp et al. 2023). A study conducted in 2010 found 95.6% seropositivity (IgG antibodies) for dengue, suggesting that most local people have been exposed to dengue infections in the past (Duncombe et al. 2013). Dengue viruses in American Samoa can be transmitted by *Aedes aegypti* and the native species *Aedes polynesiensis* (Rosen et al. 1954), which is also the vector of sub periodic lymphatic filariasis (*Wuchereria bancrofti*) (Burkot et al. 2005). CHIKV and ZIKV caused epidemics in American Samoa in 2014 (Aubry et al. 2015) and 2016 (Healy et al. 2016), respectively.

Table 4.1. Distribution of *Aedes aegypti* and *Aedes albopictus* in US states and territories. Presence reported: species has been reported at some point, but has not necessarily established local reproductive populations. Most likely established: frequent reports of a species' presence are assumed here to indicate that their populations have become locally established. Not established: these are states where these species have not established local populations.

Distribution in US and territories	*Aedes aegypti*	*Aedes albopictus*
Presence reported	Alabama, Arizona, Arkansas, California, Colorado, Delaware, Florida, Georgia, Hawaii, Illinois, Kansas, Kentucky, Louisiana, Maryland, Michigan, Mississippi, Nevada, Nebraska, New Hampshire, New Jersey, New Mexico, North Carolina, Ohio, Oklahoma, Pennsylvania, South Carolina, Tennessee, Texas, Utah, Virginia, Washington DC, Puerto Rico, US Virgin Islands, American Samoa, Northern Mariana Islands	Alabama, Arizona, Arkansas, California, Colorado, Connecticut, Delaware, Florida, Georgia, Hawaii, Illinois, Indiana, Iowa, Kansas, Kentucky, Louisiana, Maryland, Massachusetts, Michigan, Minnesota, Mississippi, Missouri, Nebraska, Nevada, New Hampshire, New Jersey, New Mexico, New York, North Carolina, Ohio, Oklahoma, Oregon, Pennsylvania, Rhode Island, South Carolina, Tennessee, Texas, Utah, Virginia, Washington, West Virginia, Washington DC, Guam, Northern Mariana Islands
Most likely established	Arizona*, California*, Florida*, Hawaii*, Louisiana, New Mexico, Texas*, Washington DC, Puerto Rico*, US Virgin Islands*, American Samoa*	Alabama, Arkansas, California*, Delaware, Florida*, Georgia, Hawaii*, Illinois, Indiana, Kansas, Kentucky, Louisiana, Maryland, Mississippi, Missouri, New Jersey, New York*, North Carolina, Ohio, Oklahoma, Pennsylvania, South Carolina, Tennessee, Texas*, Virginia, West Virginia, Guam*, Northern Mariana Islands
Most likely not established	Alaska, Colorado, Idaho, Iowa, Michigan, Minnesota, Montana, Nebraska, Nevada, North Dakota, Oregon, South Dakota, Utah, Washington, Wisconsin, Wyoming	

* Reported cases of *Aedes* transmitted viruses (2010–2024). This does not indicate which *Aedes* species was responsible for virus transmission, except in areas where only one species was present.

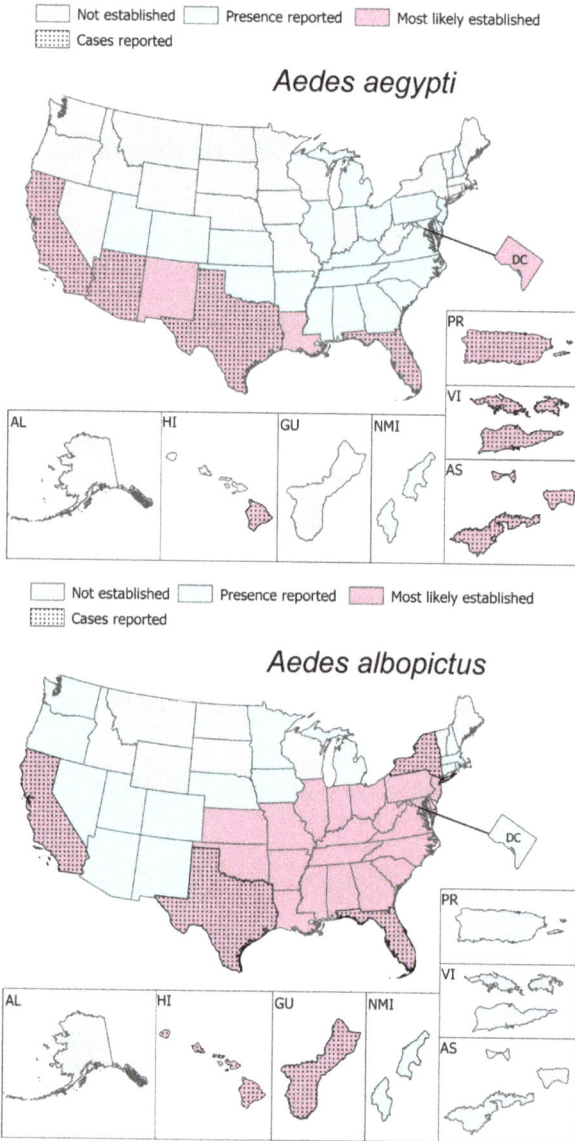

Fig. 4.1. Maps of US states and territories showing areas where *Aedes aegypti* and *Aedes albopictus* are most likely established, areas where their presence has been reported but likely not yet established, and areas where these mosquitoes are most likely not established. US states and territories with previous dengue cases (2010–2025) are highlighted, but this does not indicate which vector was responsible for transmission, except in areas where we know that only one *Aedes* species was established at the time. Al = Alaska, AS = American Samoa, DC = District of Columbia, GU = Guam, HI = Hawaii, NMI = Northern Mariana Islands, PR = Puerto Rico, and VI = US Virgin Islands. Base maps are from the US Census Bureau, https://www2.census.gov/geo/tiger/GENZ2024/shp/cb_2024_us_all_500k.zip.

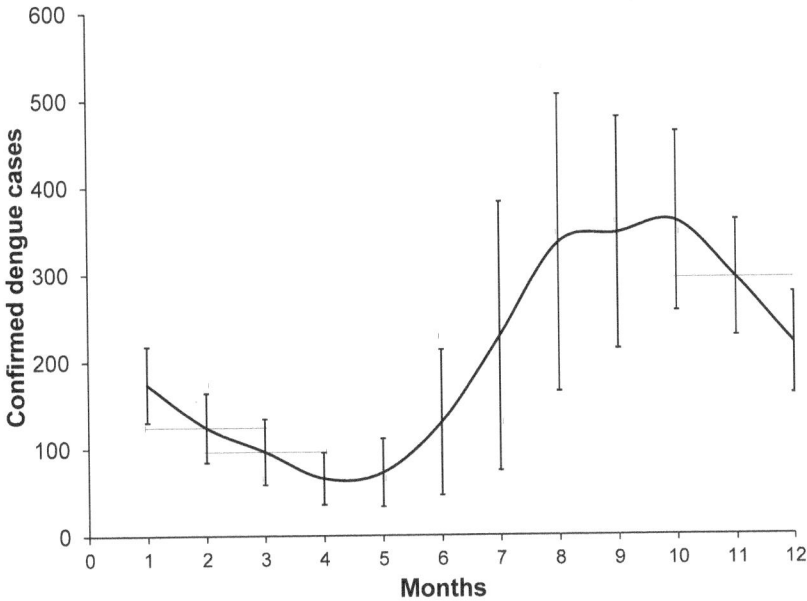

Fig. 4.2. Average (95% C.I.) number of confirmed dengue cases per month in Puerto Rico, aggregated from 1987 to 2011.

4.2. Non-endemic areas with an elevated risk of ATV emergence (*Aedes aegypti/Aedes albopictus*): Tropics/subtropics

Aedes aegypti and *Aedes albopictus* are present in multiple US states (Fig. 4.1; Table 1). Recently, ATV outbreaks have been reported in Southern Florida and Texas, while other states with subtropical climates are at risk for ATV emergence due to the presence of one or both vectors. An example is Arizona, which reported a locally acquired dengue infection in 2022 (Kretschmer et al. 2023).

Aedes aegypti keeps persistent populations in several subtropical areas of the continental US where climatic conditions allow it to survive the winter, or where vectors are frequently introduced from elsewhere. It was reported that the abundance of *Ae. aegypti* in northern Florida declined after the invasion of *Ae. albopictus*, although the former continued to be the most common mosquito species in urban areas (Omeara et al. 1995). A more recent assessment of the distribution of these species in Florida showed that *Ae. aegypti* recovered territory once occupied by *Ae. albopictus*, possibly because *Ae. aegypti* developed resistance to mating interference (Lounibos et al. 2016). The local transmission of ATVs in Texas and Florida in recent years shows that the conditions there are appropriate for dengue transmission by *Ae. aegypti* (Ramos et al. 2008, Bouri et al. 2012, Radke et al. 2012, Murray et al. 2013). Because dengue viruses are frequently introduced into these areas by infected people (Clark 2008), there is risk for local circulation in the presence of abundant *Ae. aegypti* populations.

Aedes albopictus has been repeatedly introduced into California since the early 1970s (Linthicum et al. 2003, Madon et al. 2003). Overwintering populations of *Ae. albopictus* were found in San Bernardino and Los Angeles Counties in 2002, following their initial introduction as eggs in imported lucky bamboo in 2001 (Linthicum et al. 2003). Both *Ae. aegypti* and *Ae. albopictus* have recently invaded California, spreading to eighty-five cities from 2011 to 2015 (Metzger et al. 2017). Genetic analyses traced northern and southern Californian populations of *Ae. aegypti* to southcentral US and southwestern US/northern Mexico, respectively (Pless et al. 2017). Another genetic study reported that the populations of *Ae. albopictus* in Los Angeles, California in 2011 are probably descendants from an earlier invasion in 2001, which implies that this species remained undetected for that long (Zhong et al. 2013). Two factors are expected to limit the establishment and spread of dengue vectors in southern California: (1) the local climate is usually dry during the summer and rainy during the winter, thus limiting natural mosquito productivity in rain-filled containers to the cooler part of the year (Washburn and Hartmann 1992, Moore 1999); and (2) vector control is well-organized throughout California, and this may have been a factor limiting the establishment of dengue vectors. The establishment of persistent populations of *Ae. albopictus* along the Mediterranean Sea in Europe (e.g., France, Italy, Spain) shows that this species performs well in this type of climate (Schaffner et al. 2013). Although climate is an important factor driving the dynamics of dengue vector populations, human activities strongly influence their presence and abundance. For example, a study on the distribution of *Ae. aegypti* as a function of sociodemographic factors in Los Angeles, CA found that lower income neighbourhoods had a higher abundance of this mosquito, resulting from larger backyards and abundant containers with water (Donnelly et al. 2020). The authors also found that the abundance of *Ae. aegypti* indoors was higher in neighbourhoods with less use of window and door screens and air conditioning.

Since dengue vectors have become established in California, any reported cases of ATV disease should be investigated to determine whether patients have a recent history of travel to dengue-endemic areas or it is a case of local transmission. Dengue cases reported in these states can be either imported or locally acquired, and although imported dengue cases are routinely reported in many US states, the possibility of local transmission of dengue should be investigated. Several locally acquired dengue cases were reported in Los Angeles during 2024, showing that conditions for local transmission exist in some areas of the city (CDC 2025b).

Until recently, dengue had not been reported in Hawaii since 1943/44 when both *Ae. aegypti* and *Ae. albopictus* were present (Gilbertson 1945). Similarly, there was a dengue outbreak recorded in Guam in 1944 where *Ae. aegypti* was the vector (Bailey and Bohart 1953). This species was eliminated from Guam in the following years through vector control efforts, but shortly thereafter *Ae. albopictus* invaded the islands (Reisen and Basio 1972`). There was a report to the World Health Organization of 1,418 suspected dengue cases in the Northern Mariana Islands in 2001, but it is not clear which mosquito vector was involved in that outbreak (WHO, 2025). An earlier study reported the presence of *Ae. albopictus* rather than *Ae. aegypti* in Saipan in 1991 (Mitchell et al. 1993). *Aedes albopictus* is present in several US territories in the Pacific (Guam, Northern Mariana Islands, Hawaii), where there is an increasing risk of ATV (re-)emergence. ATVs are not currently endemic in Guam, Northern Mariana Islands, or Hawaii, but ATVs have the potential to cause epidemics as illustrated by the occurrence of dengue outbreaks in Guam (2019–2021) and Hawaii (2001–2002, 2011, 2015–2016), wherein *Ae. albopictus* was the vector (Effler et al. 2005, Hasty et al. 2020).

These outbreaks illustrate that although *Ae. albopictus* is not as capable of acting as an epidemic vector of dengue as *Ae. aegypti* (Lambrechts et al. 2010), it has driven dengue outbreaks as the main vector. Detection of suspected cases in these islands should elicit an investigation to determine whether the source is travellers or ongoing local ATV transmission.

4.3. Non-endemic areas with a lower risk of *Aedes albopictus* transmission: Northern latitudes in the mainland

The distribution of *Ae. aegypti* and *Ae. albopictus* in the US has been reported and summarized by several authors (Hahn et al. 2017, Kraemer et al. 2019, Monaghan et al. 2019, Khan et al. 2020). Many records represent temporary introductions, and the surveillance of these mosquito species has been spotty in areas where ATVs have not been important. As a result, it is difficult to establish an accurate estimate of distribution (Fig. 4.1; Table 1).

Up to 2016, *Ae. aegypti* was commonly reported in Arizona, California, Washington DC, Florida, Louisiana, New Mexico, and Texas. *Aedes albopictus* was frequently reported in Alabama, Arkansas, California, Delaware, Florida, Georgia, Illinois, Indiana, Kansas, Kentucky, Louisiana, Maryland, Mississippi, Missouri, New Jersey, New York, North Carolina, Ohio, Oklahoma, Pennsylvania, South Carolina, Tennessee, Texas, Virginia, and West Virginia (Fig. 4.1; Table 1) (Hahn et al. 2017).

The discovery of an autochthonous dengue case in Suffolk County, New York in 2013 suggests the possibility of transient local DENV transmission in this temperate climate state (CDC 2025b). Dengue outbreaks were common throughout the US eastern seaboard and Gulf states from 1827 to 1941 (Ehrenkranz et al. 1971). *Aedes aegypti* was the only mosquito species involved in those outbreaks. Following introductions to an area, this mosquito species was able to undergo several generations during the summer in temperate parts of the US, or persist throughout the year at lower latitudes thanks to the presence of numerous, well-protected aquatic habitats in urban areas such as wells, cisterns, and fire-protection barrels (Chandler 1945). Currently, *Ae. albopictus* occupies much of the area originally occupied by *Ae. aegypti* and the areas further north, where it has become a nuisance mosquito with the potential to transmit ATVs.

Aedes albopictus is better adapted to persist in temperate areas than *Ae. aegypti* (Hawley 1988). Based on the observation that the distribution of *Ae. albopictus* in Asia is limited by the -5°C isotherm, it was extrapolated that this species could occupy most urban areas of the eastern US (Nawrocki and Hawley 1987). However, despite the frequent introduction of dengue viruses to those states by infected travellers, no DENV transmission had been documented until 2013 (CDC 2025b). Several factors may have prevented the occurrence of dengue outbreaks involving *Ae. albopictus* in the continental US as explained earlier, such as the use of screens in windows and doors, air conditioning, the tendency of this mosquito species to bite a variety of other vertebrates (diverting DENV into dead-end hosts), and the dependence of this mosquito on vegetated areas with low human population densities (e.g., suburban areas). Dengue cases in these states have largely been imported, particularly during the coldest months. However, as the locally acquired dengue case in New York has illustrated, the possibility of local transmission during warmer months cannot be discounted.

4.4. Areas with no risk of ATVs

There are numerous states and jurisdictions in the US where dengue vectors are absent or sporadically reported, such as Alaska, Colorado, Idaho, Iowa, Michigan, Minnesota, Montana, Nebraska, Nevada, North Dakota, Oregon, South Dakota, Utah, Washington, Wisconsin, and Wyoming (Fig. 4.1; Table 1). Although no dengue vectors have established persistent populations in these states, there is evidence of vector introductions. For example, *Ae. albopictus* was found near a tire storage facility in Ft. Lupton, Colorado in 2003, which prompted vector control measures. This species was collected again the following year, but it was not determined whether *Ae. albopictus* overwintered or if it originated from a new introduction in 2004 (Bennett et al. 2005). Further reports of this species in Colorado followed in 2005, 2010, and 2011. *Aedes aegypti* was found in Clark County, Nevada in 2017—a mosquito population that probably came from southern California (Pless et al. 2017). Other introductions of *Ae. aegypti* into higher-latitude areas of the US have been investigated, for example in Nebraska and Utah where it was found that these specimens likely originated in Southcentral or southeastern US and Tucson, Arizona, respectively (Gloria-Soria et al. 2022).

5. Dengue Vector Surveillance

This chapter underscores the necessity of monitoring *Aedes* mosquito populations to understand transmission risk, detect exotic species, and evaluate control measures. The chapter details various surveillance methods targeting both immature (larval/pupal) and adult stages, highlighting their strengths and limitations.

For pre-adults, larval indices and pupal surveys help to assess infestation levels and identify productive aquatic habitats. Adult surveillance techniques, including ovitraps, aspirators, and specialized traps like BG-Sentinel and sticky gravid traps, monitor the virus-transmitting female mosquitoes. This chapter emphasizes that adult surveillance provides a more direct measure of transmission risk.

This chapter recommends an integrated approach using both immature and adult surveillance methods. Pupal surveys inform larval control, while adult traps directly assess transmission potential. Furthermore, the chapter introduces virus surveillance in mosquitoes using RT-PCR, which indicates human infection risk and helps to pinpoint transmission foci. The vector index combines mosquito density and infection rates for a comprehensive risk assessment.

Ultimately, this chapter equips public health professionals with knowledge of essential tools and strategies for robust dengue vector surveillance, enabling data-driven interventions to reduce disease burden.

5.1. Dengue vector surveillance techniques

Vector surveillance detects the presence of and quantifies the number of mosquitoes in space and time. This is important because it can reveal if an area has been invaded by an exotic mosquito species, whether there is increased risk for virus transmission, and can measure the impact of vector control operations. It is also an essential component of ecological

    https://doi.org/10.11647/OBP.0472.05

studies that investigate the influence of weather, habitat availability, and human behaviour on vector abundance. Vector surveillance involves the use of a technique to capture mosquito specimens, followed by the identification and enumeration of specimens (in the field or laboratory), recording of data, and reporting (e.g., maps).

There are three types of data gathered during vector surveillance: the presence or absence of individuals of a particular mosquito species, the relative abundance (e.g., mosquitoes per trap per day), and the absolute abundance (e.g., mosquitoes per hectare) (Barrera 2016). Presence/absence data are most useful when the objective is eliminating the mosquito from a locality, because there is no need to count or quantify their numbers: their presence alone indicates that the species has not been eliminated. Several vector indices that are commonly used to gauge vector prevalence or to monitor the impact of control measures derive from absence/presence data (e.g., House Index). Measures of absolute population density are preferable because they capture the actual number of mosquitoes present in each area at a given time (e.g., five female mosquitoes per house), but with relative density we can compare current numbers of mosquitoes with previous or future estimates or sites (e.g., the population has doubled since the last sampling). However, the methods for obtaining accurate measures of absolute population density, such as mark-release-recapture techniques, are often too time-consuming and labor-intensive to be practical for routine mosquito surveillance in vector control programs. Effective vector surveillance requires an understanding of the ecology and behaviour of the vector species. For example, dengue vectors only lay eggs and develop their immature stages in natural and artificial *containers* with water (Fig. 5.1), not in (permanent or temporary) *pools* of water such as puddles, ponds, margins of rivers, etc. Adult dengue vectors are diurnal insects that are not attracted to conventional light traps used to capture nocturnal mosquito species (e.g., *Anopheles, Culex*). Surveillance techniques for adult dengue vectors have been limited due to the complex behaviour of these mosquitoes in response to visual, tactile, and chemical cues. For example, *Ae. aegypti* prefers biting out-of-sight on ankles and elbows to avoid humans' defensive behaviour.

Aquatic habitats of dengue vectors

Utensils (pails, tarps; paint trays)

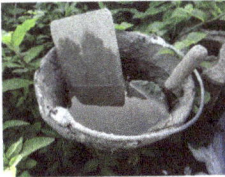

Water-storage containers (barrels, jars, tanks, cisterns)

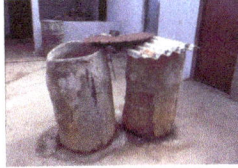

Discarded containers (tires, trash, junk)

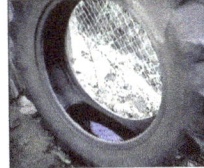

Animal drinking pans

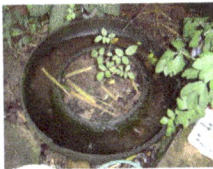

Ornamental (fountains, plant pots)

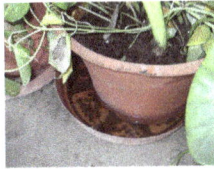

Recreational objects (plastic pools, toys, boats)

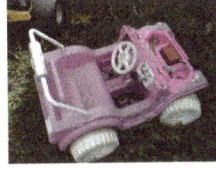

Natural containers (treeholes, bromeliads)

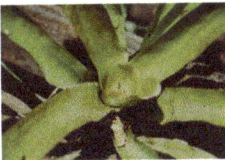

Open/broken septic tanks

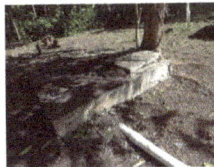

Water meters / storm drains

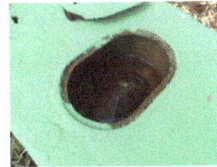

Fig. 5.1. Examples of natural and artificial containers with water used by dengue vectors to undergo immature development. Photos: CDC Dengue Branch, https://phil.cdc.gov/

The advent of new and effective traps to capture dengue vectors in their adult stages promises to advance our knowledge on the ecology and control of these mosquitoes and the viruses that they transmit. Traditional vector surveillance based on immature stages has many limitations, such as requiring intensive labour and fieldwork. Additionally, larval surveillance is less accurate and useful in estimating risk than monitoring adult mosquitoes (Focks 2003). Yet, immature surveillance is needed to understand the types of and productivity of aquatic habitats producing dengue vectors, so that more efficient, targeted control measures can be applied to productive containers. The lack of effective tools for monitoring dengue vector populations, along with the lack of clearly defined targets to assess the impact of vector control operations, may have contributed to the limited success in controlling DENV transmission worldwide.

5.2. Pre-adult mosquito surveillance

In general, it is easier to find the larvae of *Ae. aegypti* than *Ae. albopictus* or *Ae. polynesiensis*. *Aedes aegypti* is more likely to oviposit in artificial containers filled with water, while *Ae. albopictus* and *Ae. polynesiensis* more frequently utilize natural containers such as tree holes or plant axils as oviposition sites. Furthermore, there are urban areas containing cryptic aquatic habitats (e.g., wells, storm drains, sumps, roof gutters, septic tanks, elevated water tanks, service manholes) which can produce even more mosquitoes than containers that humans can identify visually (Kay et al. 2000, Montgomery and Ritchie 2002, Russell et al. 2002, Gonzalez Obando et al. 2007, Barrera et al. 2008, Pilger et al. 2011, Manrique-Saide et al. 2013). The presence of cryptic aquatic habitats for dengue vectors can only be confidently ruled out if the number of adults has significantly diminished after the control of mosquito production in containers that could be visually located (Barrera et al. 2008). Thus, the evaluation of vector control operations targeting immature mosquitoes cannot solely rely on monitoring their impact on immatures. Rather, it must include an evaluation of the impact of control measures on the adult mosquito population (e.g., before and after control).

Surveillance of immature mosquitoes relies on visual inspections of indoor and outdoor water-holding containers in buildings to check for the presence of mosquitoes at immature stages. The equipment needed to conduct immature surveillance consists of flashlights and mirrors to examine the interior of containers, and tools to examine the water and to collect mosquitoes (pan, sieve, washing bottle, suction devices to collect larvae and pupae such as a dropper or turkey basters, dippers, vials, or plastic collection bags, etc.). Large containers, such as tanks and water barrels, are sampled using sweep nets (Tun-Lin et al. 1995, Romero-Vivas et al. 2002). Inspections of underground aquatic habitats—such as wells, cisterns, and septic tanks—require the use of special devices to sample the immature stages (e.g., miniature floating funnel traps (Harrison et al. 1982, Kay et al. 1992, Russell and Kay 1999, Burke et al. 2010) or the adults emerging from such habitats when it is not possible to sample the immatures (e.g., adult emergence trap) (Barrera et al. 2008). Compound microscopes are required to identify container *Aedes* larvae and pupae. Some morphological and behavioural differences exist between the larvae and pupae of *Aedes* and other common mosquitoes inhabiting containers, such as *Culex* species. Experienced people can distinguish between these genera using bare sight. For example, the syphons of *Culex* species are longer than those of *Aedes*, and the larvae and pupae of *Culex* move faster and at wider angles than *Aedes* pupae (Fig. 5.2).

Siphons of the larvae of *Aedes* and *Culex*

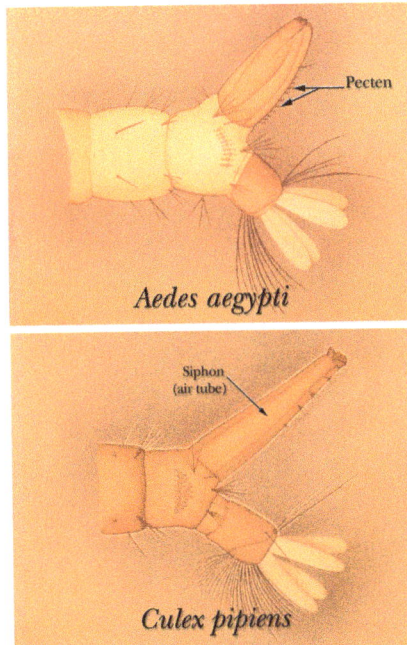

Fig. 5.2. Siphons of *Aedes* and *Culex* larvae. CDC, public domain, https://phil.cdc.gov/

The abundance and types of containers (Fig. 5.1) available to *Aedes* species need to be determined for each locality (e.g., neighbourhood), so that vector control interventions can target the most productive aquatic habitats. For example, if the most prevalent water-holding containers are discarded objects (tires, cans, etc.) on patios and lawns, it would make the most sense to emphasize source reduction efforts. This can be achieved by inspecting buildings and public areas in search of containers holding water and immature mosquitoes. It has been shown that the most productive type of container locally can be identified by inspecting less than 200 houses per neighbourhood (Barrera et al. 2006a).

5.2.1. Larval surveys (*Stegomyia* indices)

5.2.1.1. Single-larva surveys

In this type or survey, every water-holding container located in every inspected property is recorded and classified as positive if it contains immature mosquitoes, or otherwise classified as negative (Sheppard et al. 1969). A single larva per positive container is collected (usually in a vial or Whirl-Pak) and transported to the laboratory for identification. This type of survey provides data on the presence or absence of each mosquito species, and enables calculation of the House Index (HI: percentage of houses with at least one positive container), Container Index (CI: percentage of all containers with water that are positive), and Breteau Index (BI: number of positive containers per 100 houses (Connor and Monroe 1923, WHO 2009). Data from single-larva surveys do not provide information about the co-occurrence of mosquito species (e.g., *Ae. aegypti* and *Ae. albopictus*). These surveys can cover a larger area than regular surveys where all immature mosquitoes are enumerated and identified. This approach also allows the participation of personnel without training in immature mosquito identification, as they only need to collect and transport the specimens to the laboratory.

5.2.1.2. Immature surveys

These surveys involve examining all or most immature mosquitoes found in every container and recording whether they are positive or negative. The same container indices are calculated as before. In areas where *Ae. aegypti* is the only dengue vector, or if there is no interest in discerning between *Ae. aegypti* and *Ae. albopictus*, health inspectors that have been trained to recognize the larvae and pupae of these species simply record whether the container is positive or negative for *Aedes* (*Stegomyia*) species, without having to identify all the immature specimens found. The sample size needed for a reliable assessment of immature *Aedes* infestation (e.g., HI) depends on the percentage of houses that are positive. Generally, the lower the infestation, the larger the sample size (number of houses) needed. For example, in a locality with 1000 houses, if the HI is less than 1% then 258 randomly selected houses will need to be inspected; whereas if the HI is greater than 5%, only 57 houses will require inspection (PAHO 1994).

5.2.1.3. Threshold indicators for dengue transmission based on larval surveys

It has been suggested that localities with a House Index of <5% (Soper 1967), a Container Index of <10% (Connor and Monroe 1923), or a Breteau Index of <5 (Brown 1977b) are protected from yellow fever epidemics. A study in Brazil showed suppression of dengue transmission when the HI was less than 1% (Pontes et al. 2000). Some caution should be taken when interpreting these indices. 'One should not [...] predicate a critical index for a town as a whole' (Carter 1931). The reason why average values for towns are not used is that there may be areas within a town with higher indices where ATV circulation may occur.

5.2.2. Pupal surveys

5.2.2.1. Pupal demographic surveys

Pupal demographic surveys are based on the assumption that pupal productivity (pupae per person per unit time) is a better proxy for adult productivity than traditional indices (HI, CI, and BI) or larval counts (Focks 2003). Pupal populations of *Aedes* are highly correlated with the number of larvae and adults, and pupal counts can be used to estimate absolute pupal population density (e.g., pupae per hectare).

Pupal surveys are necessary to gain an understanding of what types of containers produce most of the adult *Aedes* mosquitoes, so that interventions can target those containers (Focks and Chadee 1997, Nathan and Focks 2006). Because pupae tend to aggregate such that most containers have (almost) no pupae and a few containers have many pupae, pupal surveys must sample many houses and containers to obtain a reliable estimation (Reuben et al. 1978, Barrera et al. 2006b). However, several methods have been devised to reduce the required sample size for pupal surveys (Alexander et al. 2006, Barrera et al. 2006a, Barrera 2009).

Conducting pupal surveys is like conducting larval surveys (household inspections), but only *Aedes* (*Stegomyia*) pupae are identified and counted. In the process of collecting pupae, immature indices can also be derived from presence/absence data as explained earlier. When there is more than one *Aedes* species in the area, the pupae are typically identified under a stereoscope or, alternatively, from their adult forms allowed to emerge in a controlled cage.

5.2.2.2. Threshold indicators for dengue transmission based on pupal surveys and conditions for dengue transmission

Among the relevant applications of this technique is the potential to determine threshold values of pupae per person, above which dengue outbreaks might occur. For example, models have revealed that it would take between 0.5 and 1.5 *Ae. aegypti* pupae per person to sustain dengue virus transmission at 28° C in a human population with 0–67% immunity to dengue (Focks et al. 2000). Controlled field validation of thresholds for dengue transmission based on pupal surveys has not been conducted.

5.3. Adult mosquito surveillance

Estimating the population of adult dengue vectors at a specific time and locality is important for understanding the ecological factors that affect mosquito populations, such as weather conditions, and how those factors relate to ATV transmission. It is also useful to evaluate the impact of control interventions. There are several innovations that enable reliable estimations of adult dengue vectors, contributing to a better understanding of their ecology and control. The following sections cover the various methods currently used to track adult dengue vector populations.

5.3.1. Oviposition surveys

Oviposition surveys take advantage of the fact that gravid *Aedes* females lay their eggs in artificial containers. Oviposition cups or ovitraps (Fig. 5.3) can be used to detect the presence or absence of gravid females (Fay and Eliason 1966, Reiter et al. 1991, Mackay et al. 2013). Ovitraps are small metal, glass, or plastic containers, usually of a dark colour, containing water and a rough substrate where female mosquitoes lay their eggs (wood, germination paper, cloth, cross-linked polyacrylamide) (Barrera et al. 2013a). Ovitraps can be made more attractive to mosquitoes with grass or tree leaf infusions instead of just water. Ovitraps should not be left unattended in the field for more than one week because they could start producing adult mosquitoes. These oviposition surveys can produce data on the percentage of ovitraps with eggs (positive) and the number of eggs per ovitrap.

Devices to sample dengue vector populations

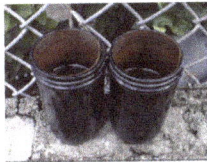

Ovitraps

Electro-mechanical aspirators

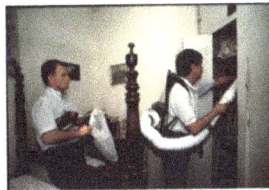

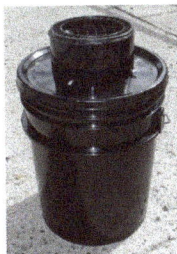

CDC Autocidal gravid ovitrap (AGO trap)

BG-Sentinel® trap

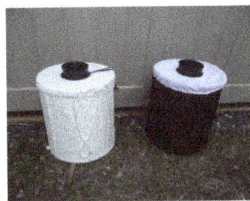

Fig. 5.3. Various devices used to collect data on adult forms of dengue vectors.
Photos: CDC, public domain, https://phil.cdc.gov/

Ovitraps are inexpensive, easy to deploy, and non-invasive, as they can be placed on the exterior of houses or properties without the need for entry. Counting the eggs requires training and a stereoscope, particularly when there is debris on the ovipositing surfaces. Collected eggs need to be hatched in the laboratory to grow the larvae until they become adults for identification purposes. This is particularly critical if more than one *Aedes* species is present.

As discussed earlier, ovitraps compete at a disadvantage with naturally occurring aquatic habitats which may be more attractive to ovipositing females, so ovitrap data may not accurately reflect the density of gravid females. Also, the values obtained following source reduction (removal of containers producing mosquitoes during control operations) might be erratic, because most extant females would find fewer water-holding containers and so would concentrate more eggs in the ovitraps (Focks 2003).

In general, fewer than 100 ovitraps are needed to obtain a reliable statistical estimate of the percentage of positive ovitraps, which serves as an indicator of the presence or abundance of mosquito species in urban areas, such as a large neighborhood (Mogi et al. 1990). Sampling sites using ovitraps, as with other mosquito traps, should not be too close together, for surveillance purposes to avoid data redundancy (two or more ovitraps reflecting the same, correlated data). As a rule of thumb, sampling sites should be 150–200m apart, assuming that such a distance is the average flight range of *Aedes* adults. Also, it has been shown that adults of *Ae. aegypti* cluster up to 30m from houses (Getis et al. 2003), so sampling sites with ovitraps should be placed at a further distance apart than that. Typically, one or more ovitraps should be placed per city block. Ovitraps are also useful for collecting *Aedes* specimens for laboratory assays, such as for insecticide resistance assays because eggs can be easily transported and stored for further analyses.

Another tool that can be used to monitor ovipositing female mosquitoes is the larvitrap. A larvitrap is a container like an ovitrap where female mosquitoes lay their eggs (e.g., a section of a tire, bamboo vase, cup) (Pena et al. 2004, Cox et al. 2007), which are then stimulated to hatch (through topping with water every week) so that developing larvae can be collected, enumerated, and identified within a week.

5.3.2. Adult mosquito surveys

5.3.2.1. Landing counts

Capturing female *Aedes* mosquitoes as they approach a human subject to bite is a highly effective technique for detecting and quantifying dengue vectors. Due to the absence of prophylactics against arbovirus infections, personnel engaged in capturing *Ae. aegypti* mosquitoes may face exposure to infective bites. Consequently, it is imperative to refrain from using this capture technique in areas where arbovirus transmission is known to occur. Other limitations of this technique are the labour involved and the variable ability of personnel to attract and collect specimens. Landing mosquitoes are collected using hand nets or aspirators. A tent trap has been developed to collect dengue vectors using human bait to protect collectors from mosquito bites (Casas-Martinez et al. 2013).

5.3.2.2. Mosquito aspirators

Mouth and electromechanical aspirators are used to collect resting mosquitoes indoors and outdoors. Mouth aspirators are not recommended for use due to the risk of aspirating pathogens that may be present on surfaces, some of which can be fatal. Electro-mechanical aspirators are safer and more efficient (Fig. 5.3) (Hayes et al. 1967, Clark et al. 1994, Vazquez-Prokopec et al. 2009). Electro-mechanical aspirators are particularly useful in collecting *Ae. aegypti* because they are 'indoor' mosquitoes, and the data from this collection technique can be used to infer mosquito density per unit area (per house, master bedroom, etc.). Sampling indoors is commonly standardized. For instance, aspiration might occur for 10–15 minutes per house. However, since aspirating mosquitoes indoors for 10 minutes only captures a small proportion of all mosquitoes, a correction factor has been proposed to estimate the total numbers of adult *Ae. aegypti* inside a house (Koyoc-Cardeña et al. 2019). The collection of adult dengue vectors outdoors is more difficult to standardize to produce comparable results. A major limitation of this useful technique is that it is labour intensive and requires trained personnel. This technique has been used to determine the impact of vector control interventions (Barrera et al. 2008). Since the number of adult mosquitoes per house largely varies, this technique requires the sampling of many houses in a short period of time (e.g., 200 houses per neighbourhood).

5.3.2.3. Passive, gravid female mosquito traps

There are several recently developed traps for collecting dengue vectors that use similar principles of attraction to ovitraps to lure and capture gravid females. These traps use either a funnel to prevent captured mosquitoes from leaving the trap (Gomes et al. 2007, Eiras et al. 2014) or a sticky glue board (Chadee and Ritchie 2010, Mackay et al. 2013, Barrera et al. 2014b). Sticky trap and ovitrap samples tend to be highly correlated, but some sticky traps have greater sensitivity at detecting dengue vectors than ovitraps (Facchinelli et al. 2007, Mackay et al. 2013). The required sample size to attain a reliable precision has been calculated for some of the sticky traps, showing that relatively few traps are required to obtain reliable estimations (Facchinelli et al. 2007, Mackay et al. 2013). Captures of female *Ae. aegypti* in CDC sticky gravid ovitraps (Fig. 5.3, CDC Autocidal Gravid Ovitraps; AGO traps) and BG-Sentinel traps are significantly correlated. The advantage of passive gravid traps is that they are considerably cheaper and easier to operate (Barrera et al. 2014b). Another important aspect of monitoring gravid females of *Ae. aegypti* is that they may be infected, because in order to produce eggs, they must have taken at least one blood meal. Several studies have used AGO traps to monitor the presence of arboviruses in *Ae. aegypti* (Barrera et al. 2017, Barrera et al. 2019a). The presence of arboviruses in *Ae. aegypti* also indicates their presence in nearby infected humans, because this mosquito does not fly very far.

5.3.2.4. Electro-mechanical traps

Adult dengue vector mosquitoes are not often captured efficiently by the most used mosquito traps, such as the CDC miniature light trap, CDC gravid trap, or New Jersey types of traps. There are several fan-operated traps designed to capture *Ae. aegypti* adults, which take advantage of the propensity of this species to be attracted to dark objects (Fay 1968,

Fay and Prince 1970, Wilton and Kloter 1985, Freier and Francy 1991). The Fay-Prince trap has been the most widely used trap, but it is heavy and bulky, making it difficult to use in sufficient numbers to achieve a reliable estimation of mosquito density.

A smaller electro-mechanical trap that uses principles of visual attraction similar to the Fay-Prince traps (white and black colour contrast) is commercially available and has the advantage of being collapsible and light in weight (Fig. 5.3, BG-Sentinel trap; Biogents, Regensburg, Germany) (Krockel et al. 2006). BG-Sentinel traps have been shown to be more effective at capturing *Ae. aegypti* than CDC backpack aspirators, and they also collect adult females in a wider range of physiological states (Maciel-de-Freitas et al. 2006, Williams et al. 2006, Ball and Ritchie 2010). These traps are also effective for collecting *Ae. albopictus* (Meeraus et al. 2008, Bhalala and Arias 2009, Farajollahi et al. 2009, Obenauer et al. 2010) and *Ae. polynesiensis* (Schmaedick et al. 2008). BG traps have been used to monitor the impact of vector control measures (Chambers et al. 2009, Rapley et al. 2009, Azil et al. 2011, Barrera et al. 2014b) and to investigate the spatial distribution and seasonal fluctuations of container-inhabiting mosquitoes (Azil et al. 2010, Barrera 2011, Barrera et al. 2011, Mercer et al. 2012). BG traps can be used with lures (e.g., CO_2, BG-Lure) to increase captures of dengue vectors. The use of octenol, an attractant for some mosquitoes, was found to decrease the number of *Ae. aegypti* in BG traps (Barrera et al. 2013b). Yields and trap sensitivity for *Ae. aegypti* and *Ae. mediovittatus* in BG traps were increased when a black outer cover was used instead of the original white one (Fig. 5.3) (Barrera et al. 2013b). Similar results were obtained using black BG traps to capture *Ae. albopictus* in Mauritius (Iyaloo et al. 2017). Eventually, the body of the BG trap was changed from white to dark blue. Williams et al. (2007) provided guidance on the number of original BG traps that should be deployed in order to attain reliable estimations of *Ae. aegypti* in Australia.

5.3.2.5. Threshold indicators for dengue transmission based on adult mosquitoes and conditions for dengue transmission

Several works have provided observational data on transmission thresholds based on ovitraps and sticky ovitraps. Significant correlations were calculated between ovitrap data and dengue incidence with time lags of up to fourteen weeks in Taiwan (Wu et al. 2013). Ovitrap data have been found to be correlated with weather and dengue incidence in Puerto Rico (Barrera et al. 2011). There were no cases of dengue haemorrhagic fever in Thailand when the density of eggs per ovitraps exposed in the field for five days was between two and fifteen (Mogi et al. 1990). Sticky ovitraps have been used for *Ae. aegypti* surveillance during a dengue outbreak in Australia, indicating that a density of two or more females per trap per week was associated with dengue cases, whereas a density of less than one female per trap per week was a safe level (Ritchie et al. 2004). Densities lower than three female *Ae. aegypti* per AGO trap per week have been shown to protect against CHIKV transmission in Puerto Rico (Sharp et al. 2019). Capturing three female *Ae. aegypti* per AGO trap per week was found to be equivalent to capturing one female per black BG trap per day (Barrera et al. 2013b). Having a well-defined mosquito density threshold provides vector control programmes with a target that relates to protection against local outbreaks of arboviruses transmitted by dengue vectors. The increasing availability and use of traps to capture adult dengue vectors will increase our knowledge on minimal mosquito densities required to prevent arbovirus transmission.

5.4. Dengue vector surveillance recommendations

Dengue vector surveillance has relied on the use of immature indices because it was very difficult to monitor the adult dengue vector population until recently. With the advent of the newer traps for adult *Aedes* (BG, sticky gravid traps), it is now possible to track the individuals that actually transmit ATVs: the female adult mosquitoes. These tools will most likely facilitate the evaluation of the impact of control measures and the establishment of entomological indicators of the risk of ATV transmission. BG-Sentinel traps are useful to perform relatively quick evaluations of changes in dengue vectors, such as before and after focal mosquito control. BG traps need to be placed in protected areas to avoid being vandalized or having their batteries stolen. Passive *Aedes* gravid traps are relatively inexpensive, sturdy, and less likely to be vandalized. They are more amenable for deployment in large numbers because they do not require power or frequent visits and are easier to operate. In addition to the use of adult traps, ovitraps have a role to play as surveillance tools with vector control programmes because they can be deployed in relatively large numbers and well-designed protocols can inform of the presence or absence of dengue vectors.

Immature surveys, and particularly pupal surveys, are needed to understand container productivity and to show the types of immature control measures that would be best adapted to the local ecology of dengue vectors. Monitoring population changes based on immature mosquitoes is time consuming and there is a risk of excluding cryptic, highly productive containers. The evaluation of immature vector control measures should involve monitoring changes in both the pupal and adult mosquito populations. In some instances, significant reductions in pupae have been observed with no change in the adult mosquito population, which indicates that key productive containers were missed (Barrera et al. 2008).

In cases where the objective is vector elimination, mosquito surveillance can concentrate on detecting the presence or absence of dengue vectors. As mosquitoes become scarcer due to vector elimination measures, they also become more difficult to detect. This calls for enhanced adult mosquito surveillance using the most sensitive types of traps available. Because BG-traps capture nulliparous, recently emerged adults, they serve as indicators of nearby aquatic habitats. On the other hand, deploying many more passive, sticky gravid traps and even ovitraps allows more widespread, continuous monitoring of the presence or absence of dengue vectors. Detection of adult mosquitoes should prompt a search for the containers producing them.

5.5. Virus surveillance in mosquitoes

Virological surveillance in mosquitoes is an important component of vector management programmes because it can indicate the threat of human infection and can be extrapolated to assess the impact of control measures. In arboviral systems such as West Nile Virus (WNV) that have zoonotic cycles, viruses circulate between wild vertebrates and mosquitoes, and virological surveillance in mosquitoes has been useful to predict the imminent risk of spillover to humans (Kilpatrick and Pape 2013). Because urban dengue viruses circulate only between mosquitoes and people, infected mosquitoes and people are bound to co-vary. In some cases, increases in mosquito infection rates have been found to precede outbreaks or heightened transmission of DENV (Chow et al. 1998, Mendez et al. 2006), but not in other cases (Chen et al. 2010). Variations in collection techniques (backpack aspirators, sweep nets, traps, human bait), sample sizes, times of the year, and human population immunity make it difficult to compare mosquito infection rates.

Reported infection rates of *Ae. aegypti* vary depending on where and when mosquitoes are captured. When mosquitoes are collected at places with known ATV cases or high-risk areas, infection rates (IRs) can be higher (1.8–57 per thousand) (Chow et al. 1998, Urdaneta et al. 2005, Garcia-Rejon et al. 2008) than in places randomly or semi-randomly sampled (0.6–2.3 per thousand) (Halstead et al. 1969, Chung and Pang 2002, Mendez et al. 2006, Chen et al. 2010, Barrera et al. 2019a). Thus, finding ATV-infected mosquitoes early in the transmission season would necessitate trapping many mosquitoes. Because dengue vectors are usually low-density mosquitoes, many sites would need to be simultaneously sampled in a short period of time to collect enough mosquitoes for dengue virus detection. A useful description of the prevalence of ATVs in dengue vectors is the vector index (VI) that reflects the expected number of infected mosquitoes, which is obtained by multiplying the infection rate by the average density of dengue vectors (Jones et al. 2011, Barrera et al. 2019a).

Monitoring dengue viruses in mosquitoes is useful to establish the likely places where humans are being infected, which is difficult to establish by other means. For example, DENV-infected *Ae. aegypti* mosquitoes were found in eleven of twenty-four schools investigated in Mexico (Garcia-Rejon et al. 2011), which underscored the importance of these sites for the transmission of DENV in the Yucatán Peninsula. Entomo-virological surveillance of *Ae. aegypti* and *Ae. albopictus* detected the presence of ZIKV in the absence of human cases in Mexico, which prompted vector control actions (Huerta et al. 2017). Furthermore, ATV cases that would not have been reported to the epidemiological surveillance system were discovered in Foz do Iguaçu City, Brazil through active serological surveillance of symptomatic cases around mosquito sampling sites following the detection of ATVs in *Ae. aegypti*

(Leandro et al. 2022). Entomo-virological surveillance in dengue vectors can complement epidemiological surveillance for ATV cases, given that community transmission may go unnoticed for some time using passive surveillance systems (Teixeira et al. 2002, Radke et al. 2012, Rowe et al. 2023). Non-endemic urban areas with established vector populations and a large influx of tourists or travellers from dengue-endemic areas may benefit from conducting periodic surveillance of ATV in mosquitoes. A comparison of virological surveillance in *Ae. aegypti* and humans during a ZIKV epidemic concluded that entomo-virological surveillance is useful to monitor epidemic activity when human surveillance is limited or when transmission intensity is low (Madewell et al. 2019).

The best method for detecting ATVs in mosquitoes will depend upon the resources available, laboratory facilities, and staff expertise. Reliable testing of specimens is an important aspect of surveillance programmes. The timeliness of this process should be stressed to alert public health officials to potential virus transmission. Currently, the most reliable technique used to detect ATVs in mosquitoes is reverse transcriptase (RT)-polymerase chain reaction (PCR). A Trioplex real-time RT-PCR assay can now detect viral RNAs of DENV, CHIKV, and ZIKV (Santiago et al. 2013, Santiago et al. 2018). Assays based on RT-PCR have the added ability to detect specific DENV serotypes. The number of PCR runs needed to detect RNA of these arboviruses can be substantially reduced by using a super pool approach. For example, aliquots or subsamples of each of ten pools are mixed in one super pool and tested. If the super pool is positive, then each of the ten pools are tested individually. On the contrary, if the super pool was negative, then no more testing is required. Because most mosquito pools will be negative due to the very small infection rates, the super pool approach can save resources and time, allowing more pools to be tested.

Viral RNA of DENVs has been detected using RT-PCR in inoculated mosquitoes that were exposed to sticky surfaces, mimicking mosquitoes captured in sticky traps under tropical field conditions for several weeks, showing that it is not necessary to restrict testing on frozen or freshly captured specimens (Bangs et al. 2007). It was shown that under laboratory conditions, ZIKV can be detected using RT-PCR in desiccated *Ae. aegypti* mosquitoes for up to thirty days (Burkhalter and Savage 2017). Another study under laboratory conditions (28°C, RH 80 ± 5%)

showed the potential to detect RNA of CHIKV using RT-PCR in *Ae. aegypti* placed on sticky tape for up to twelve weeks (Mavale et al. 2012). These results help to simplify entomo-virological surveillance efforts in locations where neither dry ice nor liquid nitrogen are readily available. However, if the task is to cultivate the virus for complete identification (e.g., genomic sequencing) rather than testing fragmented pieces of viral RNA, then collected mosquitoes should be handled following a cold chain protocol ensuring that specimens are kept frozen until analysis.

Rapid detection test devices are alternatives to laboratory-based assays that are useful for testing mosquitoes while in the field. Similar devices have been useful in detecting West Nile virus in pools of mosquitoes (Burkhalter et al. 2006, Sutherland and Nasci 2007). Dengue non-structural protein 1 (NS1) kits have proven to be useful in situations where laboratory testing is unavailable (Tan et al. 2011, Muller et al. 2012, Voge et al. 2013). A more recent development uses isothermal technique recombinase polymerase amplification lateral flow detection (RT-RPA/LFD), which allows identification of the four DENV serotypes (Ahmed et al. 2022).

6. Dengue Vector Control

Vector control is implemented in several situations: to eliminate a dengue vector species that has invaded a new area and prevent its spread; to contain an ATV that may spread following its introduction to an area (through travel, for example); to prevent outbreaks in regions where dengue vectors are already established; and to manage impending or declared dengue epidemics.

Effective vector control requires an integrated vector management programme. This programme trains vector control personnel, implements vector control activities, maintains and analyses data, produces reports, and is responsible for the efficacy of these activities. It also coordinates inter-governmental and agency collaboration, maintains liaisons with nongovernmental organizations, recommends policies and legislation, and develops educational materials for the public.

The programme should be directed by a doctoral-level professional or somebody with equivalent experience (entomologist/biologist/ecologist), with the capacity to manage all aspects of the programme whilst supported by a high-level administrator. The programme should have doctoral and master-level personnel responsible for training control personnel, supervising control activities in the field, and conducting operational research and evaluation activities, such as testing novel vector control tools. Field personnel (supervisors, inspectors) to carry out vector surveillance and control should be based within the regions (districts, municipalities). Other key personnel include health educators to develop educational and training materials for vector control professionals and the public/communities, promote community participation in vector control activities, maintain intra- and inter-agency collaboration and coordination, and interact with the press.

This chapter details strategies for effective dengue vector control. Success depends on the quality of the control agent, efficiency of the delivery system, coverage, and impact evaluation, considering the resilience of *Aedes* mosquitoes.

 https://doi.org/10.11647/OBP.0472.06

Pre-adult control targets aquatic habitats, where immature mosquitoes develop, through environmental management (eliminating containers) and larvicides (bio-rational options like Bti and Spinosad, insect growth regulators, and monomolecular films). Biological control uses aquatic predators. In order to evaluate the success of pre-adult control, both immature and adult populations should be monitored.

Adult control involves chemical methods like residual insecticide spraying (indoor/outdoor spraying, barrier treatments) and space spraying. Mosquito traps employ 'pull' strategies, such as ovitraps/ gravid traps (sticky, insecticide-treated, or larvicide-containing) or attractive toxic sugar baits (ATSBs). Mass trapping with gravid traps shows promise in reducing vector populations and disease transmission, contingent on trap efficacy and coverage.

Effective vector control necessitates an integrated approach targeting all life stages, with community involvement and continuous evaluation, due to the adaptability of dengue vectors. The selection of appropriate methods depends on the local ecology of vectors and the specific goals of the control programme.

6.1. Integrated, area-wide vector control vs focal control

Area-wide vector control is the management of the mosquito population in a whole target area, or controlling the mosquito population to levels where ATV transmission is either prevented or interrupted. Implementing control measures to an adequate spatial extent is necessary to substantially reduce the mosquito population. This involves applying control measures to entire neighbourhoods. This type of control can be used to eliminate an introduced dengue vector species, and to prevent and control ATV outbreaks.

Focal control is commonly used in response to complaints of unusual mosquito activity, to contain dengue transmission in and around areas with known cases of ATVs (e.g., 100m around the index house)—either because there is an ongoing outbreak or because ATVs have been newly introduced to the area. One limitation of focal vector control during outbreaks is that most dengue infections are asymptomatic (Endy et al. 2011, Asish et al. 2023) and difficult to detect in passive surveillance systems (based on symptomatic people seen and reported by physicians). If a large proportion of asymptomatic infections are not detected and located, this means that focal treatments would only address a small proportion of places with ongoing infections. Additionally, because the place of infection is usually unknown and thus registered as the domicile of the patient, conducting focal control around the patient's home might be unnecessary. During an epidemic, when there are large numbers of detected and reported cases, vector control programmes may not have enough resources to conduct focal control everywhere. Focal control of dengue transmission may be effective if it is applied soon after a new ATV is introduced and detected (Ritchie 2005).

6.2. Elements of successful vector control

There are four key aspects of successful vector control to be considered: control agent, delivery system, coverage, and evaluation of impact.

The control agent is used to kill the mosquitoes (e.g., pesticides, predators, traps), suppress their reproductive potential (e.g., sterile insect technique), or both (e.g., autocidal gravid traps). The effectiveness of a control agent against local dengue vectors needs to be verified (e.g., no insecticide resistance). Ideally, the longer a control agent acts (e.g., longer than the period of egg quiescence, mosquito generational time) without losing effectiveness (e.g., 100% lethality) the better, because it reduces the costs and necessary frequency of re-applications.

The delivery system is how the control agent reaches the target mosquitoes. For example, non-residual adulticides applied from trucks or aircrafts will eliminate outdoor, flying mosquitoes in the absence of insecticide resistance, if applied at the right time of the day. If most mosquitoes rest indoors, then applying insecticides outdoors is bound to have a limited impact (Reiter and Gubler 1997). In such cases, indoor spraying of insecticides is more effective, as has been reported in Iquitos, Peru (Reiner et al. 2019). To spray insecticides efficiently, spraying equipment must be calibrated, and personnel must be properly trained and supervised. In control approaches that release modified adult mosquitoes—such as the sterile insect technique (SIT), other types of genetically modified mosquitoes (GMM), *Wolbachia* suppression or replacement, etc.—the released specimens act as the control agent and the delivery system. Thus, releasing healthy, locally adapted adult mosquitoes at proper times of the day to ensure maximal survival and dispersal is key to success. Other vector control approaches that need efficient delivery systems to be effective at controlling mosquitoes involve mass trapping using a variety of means to attract and kill mosquitoes (autodissemination stations containing toxicants or biological control agents, attractive toxic bait stations, sticky gravid traps, etc.) (Barrera 2015a).

The coverage of control measures refers to the fraction of the mosquito population that is exposed to or impacted by the control agent, which does not always directly correspond to how thoroughly the control agent was delivered. For example, a whole neighbourhood can be space-sprayed using truck-mounted equipment with an effective insecticide and yet the target might be missed because indoor mosquitoes are not being impacted. However, the same methodology may be effective if applied in areas where mosquitoes are restricted to the outdoors, such as in most of the continental US where houses are screened and have air conditioning. One example of a theoretically efficient mode of delivering effective control agents which is not always successful in practice is house-to-house inspections to remove aquatic habitats and apply larvicides. This is because cryptic aquatic habitats might not be located and treated. In this case, even if all the houses in a neighbourhood were visited (which rarely happens), the impact of this control approach would be limited because a large fraction of the mosquito population was missed.

Every control measure or set of control measures needs to be evaluated, validated, and adapted to the local conditions of vector control programmes, preferably establishing the level of reduction achieved. For introduced vector or virus elimination programmes, the objective being evaluated is clear: there should not be any mosquitoes left. If the purpose of vector control is disease prevention or control, then the level of vector suppression achieved should result in a measurable decline of new virus infections.

Dengue vectors are highly resilient, with the capacity to quickly recover from population disturbances that impact vector abundance, such as vector control and droughts. This is mainly because their eggs remain viable for many months in their containers, so the total elimination of adults, larvae, and pupae at once does not prevent the area from being recolonized later by dormant/diapausing eggs. Another important aspect of the biology of dengue vectors is that they are adapted to thrive at low population densities. It has been shown that *Ae. aegypti* success is density-dependent, in that the population can achieve its maximum reproductive potential at low densities and therefore quickly recover from disturbances (Agudelo-Silva and Spielman 1984). For these reasons, the evaluation of vector control measures needs to consider the methodology of longitudinal experimental designs where vector responses are evaluated over time (Fitzmaurice et al. 2011).

Integrated vector control involves the use of two or more control agents, ideally targeting all stages of development (immature and adult mosquitoes) (PAHO 2019). The delivery system in integrated vector control requires community involvement, including residents, community/civic organizations, and government agencies, particularly at the county and district levels. An example of integrated vector control would be conducting door-to-door inspections of houses and public areas to eliminate discarded containers, treat essential containers with larvicides, and apply residual insecticides on surfaces where mosquitoes are expected to land (indoor/outdoor, on and around containers). This activity should always be preceded by planned communication efforts to inform the community about the objectives and importance of mosquito control, and what it is expected from them. Local civic organizations and governments are expected to collaborate in facilitating access to properties, collecting discarded containers, etc. Integrated, area-wide control of *Ae. albopictus* was explored in two areas of New Jersey and significant reductions in the mosquito populations were found, which varied in effectiveness between urban and sub-urban areas (Fonseca et al. 2013).

6.3. Control of pre-adult mosquitoes

6.3.1. Identification of productive containers and design of container-specific control measures

An important step in any dengue vector control operation is identifying the types, abundance, and productivity of containers producing mosquitoes, taking into account that container composition or types may vary among locations. Each type of container requires specific control measures that depend on the nature of the container and how it is used. There are five general types of containers producing dengue vectors:

1. Cavities in plants or parts of plants that accumulate water (tree holes, leaf axils of plants, etc.). For example, leaf axils of staple (e.g., taro, banana) and ornamental plants (e.g., bromeliads) can be locally abundant and can produce *Ae. polynesiensis* and *Ae. albopictus*. Interestingly, *Aedes aegypti* also uses leaf axils of ornamental bromeliads in Florida (Hribar and Whiteside 2010), which has been explained as a recent adaptation resulting from intensive mosquito control in artificial containers (Wilke et al. 2018).

2. Non-essential or disposable containers (discarded food and drink containers, used tires, broken appliances, etc.). What constitutes a disposable or non-essential container depends on the owner and their habits (e.g., hoarding tendencies).

3. Useful containers (water-storage vessels, potted plants and trivets, animal drinking pans, paint trays, toys, pails, etc.).

4. Cavities in structures (fence poles, broken bricks, uneven floors and roofs, roof gutters, air-conditioning trays, etc.).

5. Underground containers (service vessels in public areas such as storms drains, utility vaults, leaking water meters, wells, and broken/open septic tanks).

6.3.2. Control measures against immature mosquitoes

6.3.2.1. Environmental management

Whenever possible, permanent means of eliminating containers producing dengue vectors should be pursued. For example, establishing reliable supplies of piped water, having domestic garbage pickup and recycling programmes (for glass, metal, plastic, broken appliances, etc.), regulated the recycling of used tires (e.g. retaining replaced tires at the shop and shipping them away to recycling plants), and replacing septic tanks with sewerage.

Environmental sanitation works at two levels: household and community. Residents should be made aware of the life cycle of dengue vectors and how they as individuals can contribute to mosquito elimination: keeping tidy yards, servicing water-storage containers (with brushes, detergent, or bleach) and keeping them tightly closed, keeping plants in soil rather than water, servicing animal drinking pans and flower pots every week, keeping roof gutters clear of debris and water, and keeping septic tanks sealed or screened. At the community level (e.g., neighbourhood or district), the following services should be organized: pick-up and disposal of solid waste (including large items/ junk), recycling programmes (tire, trash), reliable supply of potable water, removal of artificial containers in public areas (alongside streams, abandoned lots, tire piles, etc.), planting ornamental trees that do not form cavities where water accumulates, and educating gardeners/ landscape contractors/landlords/other maintenance personnel on the life cycle and control of container mosquitoes.

6.3.2.2. Ovicides/Larvicides

There are no commercial ovicides against dengue vectors. Eggs would not be so much of a problem if larvicides lasting as long as viable eggs were used, because in this case hatching larvae would be exposed to lethal dosages of the larvicide. This key concept of control was employed during the eradication campaign of *Ae. aegypti* in the Americas when containers were sprayed with DDT: an insecticide with residual action lasting for months (Camargo 1967). An effective ovicide and larvicide can be easily made from a mixture of household bleach (Jacups et al. 2013a) and a thickening agent (Barrera et al. 2004, Mackay et al. 2015). However, like any other pesticide, household bleach would require approval from the Environmental Protection Agency (EPA) for use as a larvicide/ovicide in the US and territories.

There are several larvicides or inhibitors of adult mosquito emergence that can be used to control mosquito production in containers:

- **Bio-rational larvicides or bio-pesticides**. These larvicides have little or no impact on non-target organisms, do not accumulate in the environment, and are useful in managing dengue vector populations.

○ ***Bacillus thuringiensis israelensis or Bti.*** This is a bacterial larvicide that is highly specific for controlling mosquito larvae. Upon ingestion, parasporal crystal delta-endotoxins disrupt the larva's midgut epithelium membrane, causing death (Gill et al. 1992). Field applications of *Bti* to control dengue vectors have shown effectiveness for two to four weeks (Boyce et al. 2013). Field tests of two formulations of *Bti* showed 100% efficacy against *Ae. albopictus* for three weeks (Farajollahi et al. 2013). Various formulations of this larvicide can be applied by hand or using backpack, truck-mounted, or aerial mist sprayers (Jacups et al. 2013b, Pruszynski et al. 2017, Stoddard 2018).

○ **Spinosad**. This bio-pesticide is derived from the soil actinomycete *Saccharopolyspora spinosa* whose active ingredients, spinosyn A and D, cause involuntary muscle contractions that result in paralysis, fatigue, and death of mosquito larvae. This pesticide has a unique mode of action that makes it a valuable asset in the control of immature mosquitoes (Salgado 1998). A study conducted in a tire dump in Mexico showed that spinosad (DT formulation) was effective for ninety days (Garza-Robledo et al. 2011).

○ **Insect Growth Regulators (IGRs)**. These bio-rational insecticides interfere with physiological processes, and their effects are expressed some time after their application, during growth and development (e.g., moulting, metamorphosis). For this reason, the impact of these compounds is assessed by their capacity to inhibit the emergence of adult mosquitoes, whereas ordinary larvicides are expected to act directly on larval survival. At sublethal dosages, some adult mosquitoes emerge, but there may be delayed effects, lowering adult mosquito fecundity and reproduction (Mulla 1995).

▪ **Juvenile hormone analogues.** These products mimic the insect juvenile hormone that regulates immature mosquito growth and differentiation. An excess of exogenous, synthetic hormone analogues can therefore partially or totally inhibit metamorphosis, leading to the retention of old epidermal structures in the next instar.

☐ **S-methoprene.** This IGR is highly effective against dengue vectors, has low toxicity, and poses little risk to humans and other non-target species, with the exception of estuarine invertebrates (EPA 2025a, Braga et al. 2005). S-methoprene has been delivered as ultra-low volume (ULV) truck spray targeting aquatic habitats of *Ae. albopictus*, causing significant reductions in the number of mosquito adults (Bibbs et al. 2018).

☐ **Pyriproxyfen.** This juvenoid inhibits the emergence of adult dengue vectors, at very low doses. Numerous studies have investigated pyriproxyfen as a control agent against dengue vectors using manual application, ULV spraying and thermal fogging, bed nets, and candles among other modes of delivery, with varying success (Hustedt et al. 2020).

■ **Chitin synthesis inhibitors**. These products inhibit cuticle deposition, killing larvae during ecdysis (moulting) or in the pupal or adult stage.

☐ **Diflubenzuron.** This chitin synthesis inhibitor has been shown to have potential for the control of *Ae. albopictus* in Florida (Ali et al. 1995). Like other IGRs, diflubenzuron has low mammalian toxicity and little effect on non-target organisms. A tablet formulation of diflubenzuron provided 90–100% inhibition of *Ae. aegypti* emergence for ten weeks under semi field conditions (Saleh et al. 2013).

☐ **Novaluron**. Tests conducted in clay jars and pails in Thailand showed adequate control of *Ae. aegypti* after ninety days of this treatment (Mulla et al. 2003). Novaluron inhibited the emergence of temephos-resistant *Ae. aegypti* for several weeks in simulated field conditions in Brazil (temephos is an organophosphate insecticide extensively used as a larvicide to which *Ae. aegypti* has developed resistance in many countries; Fontoura et al. 2012). These researchers found reduced activity of novaluron in containers exposed to the sun. The impact of novaluron on the mortality of immature *Ae. aegypti* and *Ae. albopictus* has been demonstrated under field conditions using the product in autocidal gravid ovitraps (AGO traps) that were placed inside and outside homes in Gampaha, Sri Lanka (Withanage et al. 2020).

- **Monomolecular films and oils**. These products spread on the surface of water, forming a thin film that can cause immature mosquitoes to suffocate by preventing gas exchange. One advantage of these products over others is that they can kill both mosquito larvae and pupae. Monomolecular films are biodegradable and are relatively safe for non-target invertebrates and vertebrates (Nayar and Ali 2003). Because these products kill immatures by physical rather than chemical means, they are not expected to cause the evolution of resistance and could be used as complementary, non-chemical control agents for the management of insecticide resistance. A combination of a monomolecular film and methoprene has been shown to cause a 95% reduction in adult *Ae. albopictus* emergence in the field for thirty-two days (Nelder et al. 2010). Monomolecular films are used along with *Bti* to control immature *Ae. aegypti* in the Florida Keys, because unlike *Bti*, monomolecular films can kill pupae (Hribar et al. 2022).

Larvicides and IGRs have been used in ovitraps and gravid traps to increase the safety of these devices by preventing the production of mosquitoes inside the traps. Results from a study in Puerto Rico showed that the attraction of *Ae. aegypti* to AGO traps was not altered by the use of *Bti*, spinosad, nor novaluron (Acevedo et al. 2021).

6.3.2.3. Biological control

The use of aquatic predators to control immature dengue vectors faces several limitations. Natural and artificial containers are typically small habitats with limited external supplies of organic matter coming from decaying plant materials, occasional drowned insects, and resulting micro-organisms that do not support a diverse community of aquatic predators. Due to their small size, these habitats also suffer frequent disturbances, such as desiccation, which prevent the accumulation of predators.

Several invertebrate and vertebrate predators have been used to control immature dengue vectors, mainly cyclopoid copepods, *Toxorhynchites* mosquitoes, dragonfly nymphs, larvivorous fish, and turtles. Copepods are tiny crustaceans present in many types of aquatic habitats, including natural and artificial containers, for as long as they can last without drying out. Several copepod species are efficient predators of early instars of mosquitoes, particularly of container *Aedes* species (Marten and Reid 2007). Copepods have been used within integrated, combined vertical and horizontal community-based control programmes in Vietnam, which achieved local elimination of *Ae. aegypti* by a combination of source reduction, container recycling, and seeding copepods in water-storage containers (Nam et al. 1998). This methodology was later expanded and *Ae. aegypti* and *Ae. albopictus* were eliminated from many communes where dengue transmission was reported to cease (Kay and Nam 2005). Sustained, local elimination of *Ae. albopictus* in tire piles was also achieved in Louisiana using copepods (Marten 1990).

The larvae of *Toxorhynchites* spp. mosquitoes prey upon larvae of other mosquitoes and aquatic insects, and the adults are not hematophagous; they only feed on flower and fruit nectars. These predatory mosquitoes are also container mosquitoes (tree holes, bamboo internodes, and artificial containers), like dengue vectors. These mosquitoes are easy to rear in the laboratory and have been used to control dengue vectors on numerous occasions (Focks 2007). One important limitation for using *Toxorhynchites* as a control agent is that their adults are limited to areas with shade and vegetation where they overlap with *Ae. aegypti* and *Ae.*

albopictus, and would not be effective in the core of urban areas without vegetation or shade, where *Ae. aegypti* is the main container mosquito.

Dragonfly larvae are aquatic predators that can be used as biological control agents against several immature mosquito species including *Ae. aegypti*, *Ae. albopictus*, and *Culex quinquefasciatus* (Sebastian et al. 1990, Ramlee and Mohd 2022).

Larvivorous fish are also commonly used predators to control dengue vectors, particularly in large containers that do not frequently desiccate, such as water tanks, cisterns, ornamental fountains, etc. Species of larvivorous fish used for mosquito control should be native, have a preference for mosquito larvae, and be adaptable to confined spaces (Chandra et al 2008). Biological control agents are suited for use in community participation programmes because these agents require human care to survive in the containers in which they are seeded. An example is the Monte Verde project in Honduras, which integrated copepods, turtles, tilapia fish, and larvicides in a community participation project that showed effectiveness against *Ae. aegypti* (Marten et al. 2022).

6.3.3. Evaluation of the effectiveness of pre-adult mosquito control

The effectiveness of pre-adult mosquito controls applied in the field is usually assessed by comparing the presence/absence or abundance of immatures in treated containers before and after treatment, or by comparing with untreated areas (Chadee 2009). In the latter case, it is advised to conduct preliminary surveys to quantitatively select comparable sites. Although it is necessary to verify controls acting at immature stages, the goal is to determine the impact of control measures on the adult, biting mosquito population. Thus, in addition to immature surveillance, it is necessary to determine the level of reduction in female adult mosquitoes (Barrera et al. 2008). This is particularly important if there are highly productive, cryptic aquatic habitats that were not located and impacted (Pilger et al. 2011). If there are cryptic aquatic habitats producing dengue vectors, assessing immature reduction only in those containers that can be visually located will lead the efficacy of control measures to be overestimated, placing the human population at risk.

6.4. Control of adult dengue vectors

6.4.1. Chemical control

The chemical control of adult mosquitoes must assure contact between the insecticide and adult dengue vectors by: (1) using certain surfaces sprayed with residual insecticides where mosquitoes are expected to land; (2) actively diffusing small droplets of concentrated insecticide in the air, so that they impact the body of the mosquito while flying or resting; and (3) delivering insecticides to adult mosquitoes via ingestion of toxic baits, as presented later in relation to their use in trap devices.

Residual insecticides should be used on surfaces that adult mosquitoes frequently visit and land on, such as dark walls, closets, under furniture, in containers with water and adjacent surfaces, vegetation, and other outdoor resting sites. Indoor residual spraying (IRS) is more appropriate for controlling *Ae. aegypti* in areas where this species rests indoors, encompassing dengue-endemic areas. IRS applied to entire walls, ceilings, and furniture is not commonly used by vector control programmes in the US to control dengue vectors. Targeted IRS against *Ae. aegypti*, which involves applying a residual insecticide only on wall surfaces below 1.5m and under furniture, showed similar effectiveness to classic IRS in Mexico (Dunbar et al. 2019). The effectiveness of indoor or outdoor residual insecticide spraying against dengue vectors would benefit from more knowledge about their resting sites (Facchinelli et al. 2023). The Pan American Health Organization (PAHO) released updated guidelines for the control of *Ae. aegypti* in urban areas using indoor residual spraying (PAHO 2019).

Residual insecticide impregnated materials such as curtains and covers for water storage vessels have been investigated as tools to reduce *Ae. aegypti* populations (Kroeger et al. 2006, Vanlerberghe et al. 2011, Lorono-Pino et al. 2013). Covers for water barrels impregnated with a residual insecticide (DDT) were first used in Guam in 1945 (Bailey and Bohart 1953). Insecticide treated screening (ITS), which consists in screening a house using insecticide-treated screens, showed high effectiveness at reducing the indoor population of *Ae. aegypti* in Mexico (Manrique-Saide et al. 2021). Another type of device using residual insecticides is lethal ovitraps, where a strip with insecticide is placed as a landing surface for females seeking a place to lay eggs (Perich et al. 2003).

The barrier spraying of residual insecticides on external walls of houses and vegetation has been used effectively to reduce exposure to exophilic mosquito species (Anderson et al. 1991, Perich et al. 1993, Cilek 2008), including *Ae. albopictus* (Trout et al. 2007). Because dengue vectors in the continental US are mostly exophilic mosquitoes, it is likely that barrier treatments can also have significant effects on *Ae. aegypti*. The impact of barrier spraying residual insecticides on *Ae. aegypti* has not been explored in tropical areas where this mosquito is predominantly endophilic, but because this mosquito must regularly visit the peri-domestic environment in search of containers for egg laying, this technique might still prove useful.

Insecticides can also be space-sprayed with backpack-, truck-, or aircraft- mounted equipment. However, space spraying insecticides from the streets or air has been ineffective for controlling *Ae. aegypti* in dengue-endemic areas where this mosquito predominantly rests indoors (Reiter and Gubler 1997). The main reason for failure is that the insecticide droplets do not reach the concealed sites where this mosquito rests, such as closets, behind furniture, etc. When applied inside the home, insecticides can be effective in temporarily reducing adult *Ae. aegypti* numbers (Perich et al. 1992, Mani et al. 2005). However, this is not practical in many countries due to difficulties gaining access to the interior of homes. Space spraying using truck-mounted equipment and a novel adulticide caused significant reductions in the number of adult *Ae. albopictus* in New Jersey even when applied at night (Farajollahi et al. 2012). This method could also be useful for temporary reductions of *Ae. aegypti* in CONUS given that this mosquito species is mainly an outdoor species because the indoor environment is protected with screens.

6.4.2. Mosquito traps

Three main strategies to control dengue vectors with traps are: (1) pull (attract/kill), which refers to the strategy whereby mosquitoes are drawn to containers for oviposition (such as ovitraps and gravid traps) and are subsequently eliminated through various methods; (2) push (repel) – pull (attract/kill) consists in repelling adult mosquitoes from indoor environments while capturing those that are repelled using adult traps placed around the property; and (3) pull (attract/contaminate/infect) – push (fly away), which involves attracting adult mosquitoes without eliminating them—instead, the mosquitoes become contaminated or infected with an insect pathogen upon contact with the device. Afterward, the mosquitoes fly away, potentially interacting with other adult mosquitoes (e.g., during mating) or aquatic habitats (e.g., for oviposition), and so the contaminant or pathogen is anticipated to reduce the population of immature mosquitoes (Barrera 2022).

Pull (attract/kill)

Two main approaches are used in this category: (1) attracting gravid females to containers with water and other attractants (ovitraps/gravid traps), in which the females are eliminated; and (2) attracting mosquitoes to sugar bait stations where they ingest a lethal dose of a toxicant (attractive toxic sugar baits: ATSBs).

There are at least three types of mosquito ovitraps that have been developed and tested for the purpose of controlling *Ae. aegypti*: sticky gravid ovitraps (Ritchie et al. 2003, Ritchie 2005, Chadee and Ritchie 2010, Mackay et al. 2013, Barrera et al. 2014a, Barrera et al. 2014b, Barrera et al. 2017, Barrera et al. 2019a, Barrera et al. 2019c, Juarez et al. 2021, Barrera 2022), residual-insecticide impregnated ovitraps (Perich et al. 2003), and standard ovitraps treated with larvicides (Regis et al. 2008). Ovitraps are dark containers with water and some sort of oviposition attractant. Female mosquitoes are lured into these traps by decomposing organic materials such as hay or dry tree leaves. Insecticidal ovitraps are not recommended because they can worsen the already existing problem of insecticide resistance in dengue vectors (Johnson et al. 2018). Small ovitraps need to be attended weekly to avoid producing mosquitoes, although ovitraps can contain certain larvicides (Bti, spinosad), insect growth regulators (S-methoprene, novaluron), or yeast interfering-RNA that do not discourage oviposition (Acevedo et al. 2021, Hapairai et al. 2021, Barrera 2022). One shortcoming of small ovitraps is that they can be toppled by wind and animals.

Sticky ovitraps have the advantage of not using pesticides, so they are a useful alternative for controlling dengue vectors in areas with insecticide resistance, or they can be used in conjunction with insecticidal measures. The continuous use of mass trapping with AGO traps for several years did not cause behavioural avoidance in *Ae. aegypti* in Puerto Rico. Several studies have showed the effectiveness of mass-trapping with gravid traps in reducing: *Ae. aegypti* numbers (Barrera et al. 2019c, Ong et al. 2020, Juarez et al. 2021), infected mosquitoes (Barrera et al. 2019a), and human infections with CHIKV (50%) (Sharp et al. 2019) and DENV (36%) (Ong et al. 2020). Mass-trapping can also significantly decrease the density of *Ae. aegypti* around a target building (Barrera et al. 2018). Mass-trapping gravid females of *Ae. aegypti*: (1) reduces the number of biting mosquitos most likely to be infected because, to have become gravid, females must have taken a blood meal which could have been infective; (2) shortens the average longevity of the biting mosquito population, which may also reduce their chances to become infective; and (3) reduces the fecundity of the population (Lega et al. 2020).

The effectiveness of mass mosquito trapping depends on several factors such as trap efficiency in attracting and retaining gravid female mosquitoes, deploying the correct number of traps per unit area or building (e.g., three traps per home), achieving wide areal coverage (e.g., over 60% of houses in a neighbourhood), long servicing periods to refresh the traps—depending on the size and capacity of the trap to retain water and attractants (e.g., several weeks/months)—timely and thorough trap servicing, and acceptance from the community (Barrera 2022). It is also important to use electronic devices and GIS software to collect data, update the location and condition of the traps, and conduct quality control. Given that mass trapping requires many traps to be deployed, it is necessary to have a system to monitor their location and status, because broken traps could produce mosquitoes if left unattended. Mass-trapping, like other dengue vector control approaches, benefits from community involvement (Johnson et al. 2018).

Attractive toxic sugar baits (ATSB) lure and kill dengue vectors either when sprayed on vegetation or when used as a component of a bait station (Barrera 2022). Several toxicants have been used in ATSB, such as clove oil, garlic oil, boric acid, fipronil, and ribonucleic acid interference or RNAi, among others (Xue et al. 2008, Mysore et al. 2020). ATSBs have been shown to reduce adult populations of *Ae. albopictus* in Florida (Naranjo et al. 2013, Revay et al. 2014). Evidence is being collected to determine if these toxic baits would work against *Ae. aegypti* in tropical urban areas, because it has been reported that females of this species do not commonly consume sugars (Costero et al. 1998). However, a study in Bamako, Mali showed effective control of *Ae. aegypti* after vegetation was sprayed with a formulation of micro-encapsulated garlic oil (Sissoko et al. 2019). Another study conducted under laboratory and limited field trials showed that adults of *Ae. aegypti* can be attracted using a visual cue and killed using a dry ATSB in Machala, Ecuador (Sippy et al. 2020).

Push (repel) – pull (attract/kill)

This approach uses a spatial repellent such as transfluthrin (a volatile synthetic pyrethroid) to create a space that prevents mosquitoes from entering or staying (i.e., pushing them away) in the protected area, and uses traps to capture adult mosquitoes in the periphery of the house (i.e., pulling them). It has been reported that the push component worked better at protecting people than the push/pull combination against *Ae. aegypti* (Tambwe et al. 2020, 2021). Although repellence is involved, the volatile insecticide seems to interfere with the normal behaviour of the mosquito (e.g., biting, flying) or kill it at high concentrations. The impact of a commercially available spatial emanator placed in houses to control DENV and ZIKV transmission was evaluated using a cluster randomized trial in Iquitos, Peru (Morrison et al. 2022). This study reported reductions in ATV infections (34.1%), *Ae. aegypti* abundance (28.6%), and mosquito blood-feeding rates (12.4%).

Pull (attract/contaminate/infect) – push (fly away)

This approach involves attracting adult mosquitoes to an auto-dissemination device where the mosquitoes are contaminated with a product, which is then passed on to other adult mosquitoes (e.g., through mating) or to aquatic habitats (e.g., through oviposition). The most commonly used product in auto-disseminating devices is pyriproxyfen, as described earlier: an insect growth regulator that inhibits the immature development of mosquitos at very low dosages. Results of field trials on the effectiveness of this approach report mixed results. A long-term study aiming to use this approach to control *Ae. albopictus* in

New Jersey neighbourhoods did not result in effective mosquito control (Unlu et al. 2020). A cluster randomized trial conducted in Brazil to control *Ae. aegypti* reported significant reductions of adult mosquitoes but no changes in the number of eggs/ovitrap or trap positivity (Garcia et al. 2020). This approach, like other emerging technologies to control dengue vectors, will need to be assessed based on its impact on ATV transmission (Barrera 2022).

The World Health Organization put together guidelines for the efficient testing of traps to control dengue vectors and disease transmission (WHO 2018). This publication offers guidance through the development and testing processes, covering laboratory studies, small-scale field testing, large-scale entomological field trials, and community trials of impact on disease.

6.4.3. Biological control of adult mosquitoes

The biological control of adult mosquitoes uses living organisms to reduce the populations of mosquito vectors to levels below the threshold for the transmission of pathogens to humans or other vertebrates. It may also involve modifying the capacity of the mosquito population to transmit ATVs rather than reducing their numbers.

- **Entomopathogenic fungi.** *Metarhizium anisopliae* and *Beauveria bassiana* are being explored as biocontrol agents against dengue vectors. Mosquitoes attracted to surfaces bearing fungus conidia become infected by tarsal contact, enabling spores to attach and penetrate the cuticle, grow, and produce toxins that kill the mosquito. The longevity of adult *Ae. aegypti* and *Ae. albopictus* infected with *M. anisopliae* can be significantly reduced (Scholte et al. 2007). Reducing the longevity of female mosquitoes can significantly decrease virus transmission, because the viruses might not have enough time to disseminate and reach the salivary glands (extrinsic incubation period) that would render the mosquito infectious (Knols et al. 2010).

- **Genetically modified mosquitoes (GMM).** There are two basic approaches to control vectors through genetic modification:

(1) population suppression to reduce or eliminate the local vector population by suppressing their reproductive capacity, and (2) population replacement to eliminate the capacity of the mosquitoes to transmit a pathogen. In the first case, males are released into the environment to copulate with wild females and act as sterilizing agents, so that no viable progeny is produced or, if viable progeny develops, the mosquitoes die before reproducing. This approach requires sustained releases until the population is brought under control or eliminated (self-limited method). Classical sterile insect technique (SIT) using irradiated, sterile males falls into this category (Bellini et al. 2013). Another example is the patented, genetically modified *Ae. aegypti* carrying a dominant lethal gene (RIDL) that is currently being tested in the field (phase 3: staged open field releases) as a strategy for population suppression in several countries (Wise de Valdez et al. 2011, Alphey et al. 2013). RIDL males carrying the genetic modification mate with wild females, and the progeny carry a gene that expresses in late larval instars and causes death in the absence of tetracycline. The second approach involves introducing a genetic modification that is sustained within the mosquito population, usually aimed at making the mosquitoes resistant to pathogen transmission. This approach is said to be self-sustaining, and the idea is to replace a vector population with a non-vector population of the same mosquito species (Franz et al. 2014).

- **Endosymbiont bacteria.** This control approach involves using certain strains of *Wolbachia* endosymbiont bacteria. Some *Aedes* species such as *Ae. albopictus* naturally carry these bacteria, whereas *Ae. aegypti* does not. In the latter case, transfection has been conducted to produce *Ae. aegypti*'s infected strains. There are two main approaches being tested in a similar way as with GMM: population suppression and population replacement.

    o In the first approach, infected males are released to mate with wild females, and due to their induced cytoplasmic incompatibility there is no fertile progeny. This method necessitates that no females are released along with males, because mating between *Wolbachia*-infected males and females would produce viable progeny infected with the bacteria, leading to the establishment of the introduced strain with *Wolbachia*. If that happens, then the initial suppression approach would no longer be viable. This control method has been tested with *Ae. aegypti*, as well as with *Ae. albopictus* and *Ae. polynesiensis* (O'Connor et al. 2012). Advances in the mass production of dengue vectors have made it possible to release millions of male *Ae. aegypti* adults in a single week (Crawford et al. 2020). A pilot study conducted in three neighbourhoods of Fresno, California released 14.4 million male *Ae. aegypti*, causing a reduction of 95% of the mosquito population (Crawford et al. 2020). Another study conducted in South Miami, Florida showed a maximum suppression of adult *Ae. aegypti* by 75% (Mains et al. 2019). A similar project conducted in Ponce City, Puerto Rico achieved 50% suppression of the local *Ae. aegypti* population (Sánchez-González 2025).

○ The second approach seeks to release male and female mosquitoes carrying a *Wolbachia* strain that blocks the transmission of ATVs, in order to replace the local dengue vector population with a *Wolbachia*-infected population. This approach is being tested in several countries with transfected *Ae. aegypti*, whereby the wild population is being replaced with the infected strain after successive releases (Hoffmann et al. 2011). A cluster randomized trial was conducted in Yogyakarta, Indonesia to test the hypothesis that replacing the original *Ae. aegypti* population with one infected by a dengue-blocking strain of *Wolbachia* would reduce dengue cases (Utarini et al. 2021). The results showed a protection efficacy of 77.1% and 86.2% against virologically confirmed dengue cases and incidence of hospitalization, respectively. Follow up studies reported 78% lower incidence of dengue haemorrhagic fever in areas where the population replacement with *Wolbachia*-infected mosquitoes had reached 80–100% prevalence as compared to areas with 0–20% prevalence (Indriani et al. 2023).

Control methods that rely on the release of conspecifics to achieve population suppression or replacement (with a non-vector population) face some challenges (Barrera 2015).

- *Aedes aegypti* and *Ae. albopictus* have a limited dispersal capacity (a few hundred meters), which necessitates that release stations be close together (e.g., 2.3 release station per hectare). This could translate to hundreds or thousands of release stations in urbanized areas.

- The spatial dispersal of these mosquitoes is over-dispersed or aggregated in space, which necessitates larger release rates compared to randomly dispersed populations. Because the spatial pattern of dispersal of these mosquitoes can change seasonally, close monitoring of these populations over time is advised. The heterogeneity of the target population is an important factor.

- The capacity of *Ae. aegypti* eggs to withstand desiccation for months inside containers gives this species high resistance and resilience that requires sustained control efforts for months.

- The degree of suppression or modification of these *Aedes* species needs to impact a high percentage of the mosquito population. Lowering the density of animal species such as these mosquitoes that are under density-dependent regulation (limited by food/spatial resources or competition for these resources) may not have a large impact on their dynamics, because individuals perform well at low population densities.

- Immigration of mosquitoes from nearby, untreated areas could repopulate mosquito populations in treated areas. The use of buffer control zones around treated areas may be needed to reduce the impact of immigration (e.g., expanding control outside the target control area).

- Because several of the *Aedes* control approaches using released conspecifics are relatively recent, there is a need to document their sustainability, cost, and effectiveness.

6.4.4. Insecticide resistance and management

Dengue vectors have evolved resistance against almost every class of insecticide, including microbial pesticides and IGRs (Brogdon and McAllister 1998). Insecticide resistance occurs when there is a significant reduction of susceptibility to an insecticide that used to be effective against a dengue vector. Insecticide resistance is inheritable and results from the process of natural selection whereby the insecticide kills some individuals (susceptible) but allows other (resistant) mosquitoes to survive and reproduce. Mosquitoes may survive the action of insecticides because the insecticide cannot bind to its target (target-site resistance), or because they have enzymes that prevent the insecticide from reaching its target site (enzyme-based resistance) (Brogdon and McAllister 1998). Mosquitoes can also avoid being killed by the insecticide through behavioural avoidance, either after contact with the insecticide (irritancy) or by avoiding contact with sprayed surfaces in the first place (non-contact spatial repellent). For example, a study has found that 59% of resistant *Ae. aegypti* mosquitoes would not enter a hut sprayed with DDT, showing that DDT acts as a chemical screen (space repellence) for these mosquitoes (Grieco et al. 2007). There may also be cuticular resistance involved in insecticide resistance, where there is reduced penetration of the insecticide through the cuticle (Namias et al. 2021).

Insecticide resistance can be evaluated in the laboratory and under field conditions. In the former, field-collected mosquitoes are tested after exposure to diagnostic concentrations of an insecticide and their mortality is evaluated over time in comparison with a fully susceptible strain of the mosquito (WHO 2016, CDC 2020, Corbel et al. 2023). Results from these assays are useful to monitor changes in insecticide resistance over time and space, but they provide little information about the actual effect on dengue vectors in the field where commercial formulations are used rather than their active ingredients in isolation. Depending on the mode of delivery of the insecticide (ULV, indoor/outdoor residual insecticide applications, insecticide-treated materials, etc.), field assays should be curated to evaluate the impact on mosquito populations and vector-borne diseases (Namias et al. 2021).

Numerous studies have documented insecticide resistance in dengue vectors, particularly in *Ae. aegypti*. Resistance to pyrethroid insecticides in *Ae. aegypti* has been reported in several US states (McGregor and Connelly 2021, Wang et al. 2022), Puerto Rico (Hemme et al. 2019, 2022), and the US Virgin Islands (Kenney et al. 2017), but to a lesser extent in *Ae. albopictus* (Marcombe et al. 2014). An investigation of insecticide resistance in thirty-seven *Ae. aegypti* and forty-two *Ae. albopictus* populations in Florida (2016–2018) found that 95% of the populations of the former and 30% of the latter species were resistant to pyrethroids (Parker et al. 2020). The authors also found that 31% of the populations of both species were resistant to organophosphate insecticides. Resistance to temephos (a chemical organophosphate larvicide no longer used in the US) and pyrethroids is widespread in the Americas and Southeast Asia (Ranson et al. 2010). Resistance to pyrethroids is widespread in Mexico as a result of their sole and continued used for over ten years (Flores et al. 2013). In Brazil, insecticides have been rotated in time based on the evolution of resistance in *Ae. aegypti*, first from organophosphates to pyrethroids and back to organophosphates. Also, the evolution of resistance to temephos led to a change from chemical larvicides to *Bti*, then to diflubenzuron, and more recently to novaluron. Resistance to temephos and pyrethroids seems widespread in Latin America (Rodríguez et al. 2007). These observations underscore the need to monitor insecticide resistance in vector control programmes, illustrating how dynamic evolutionary resistance can be.

Insecticide resistance management seeks to delay or prevent the development of resistance levels before the insecticide becomes ineffective. Resistance management can be achieved by following various procedures: (1) limiting the use of insecticides to areas with the highest transmission rates—this strategy allows susceptible mosquitoes to disperse from neighbouring sites into the treated areas, thus diluting resistance; (2) rotating insecticides with different modes of action; (3) using non-chemical means of vector control in conjunction with insecticides; (4) avoiding slow degrading insecticides; (5) conducting seasonal application if other means of vector control are available for the rest of the year (e.g., source reduction, biological control); (6) using mixtures of insecticides that do not cause cross resistance; and (7) using synergistics that inhibit specific detoxification enzymes.

7. Dengue Vector Management in Dengue Outbreaks

This chapter focuses on dengue vector management during outbreaks in both endemic and non-endemic regions. In *non-endemic areas*, rapid response to imported cases is key. This should involve intensive surveillance, contact tracing, and focused vector control (residual insecticide spraying, larvicide, source reduction) within a 100m radius. High coverage is crucial for containment. Recommendations include thorough investigation of suspected cases, proactive case finding, enhanced entomological surveillance with GIS, and comprehensive, neighbourhood-wide vector control targeting breeding sites and adult mosquitoes, alongside public education.

In *endemic/epidemic areas*, controlling widespread outbreaks is challenging. Prevention through pre-emptive vector control in high-risk 'hot spot' neighbourhoods during low transmission seasons is favourable. The response should involve multi-agency collaboration, mass spraying, public education, and enhanced case management. Early warning systems can provide lead time. Sustained, integrated vector control, guided by robust surveillance and defined mosquito density thresholds, is essential.

For an epidemic response, activating an emergency operations centre is recommended. This should emphasize community education, bed net use, healthcare training, enhanced surveillance with GIS, and prioritized, area-wide vector control combining larvicide, adulticide, and source reduction. It is vital to evaluate the impact of these interventions.

Key messages for dengue prevention target behavioural changes in terms of container management and personal protection for residents and travellers, with specific advice tailored for both endemic and non-endemic areas, as well as secondary prevention within households.

©2025 Roberto Barrera, CC0   https://doi.org/10.11647/OBP.0472.07

7.1. Non-endemic areas

ATVs outbreaks in non-endemic areas may go unnoticed for a while before being detected. There is some opportunity to detect early, secondary cases arising from the index case at places where ATVs are regularly introduced by travellers, if local health authorities have an active surveillance system in place (Hills et al. 2002, Ritchie et al. 2002). The following actions were implemented in response to the detection of DENV introductions in North Queensland, Australia, where *Ae. aegypti* is present but dengue is not endemic: an outbreak was declared, dengue case surveillance was intensified, follow-up case interviews were conducted to identify potential infection sites, and sustained dengue vector control measures were enacted to contain the virus and prevent its spread to other urban areas. Additionally, an educational programme was maintained to raise awareness about dengue, explaining how the virus is transmitted and encouraging residents to take proactive measures to control dengue vectors in their homes.

During a dengue outbreak in Cairns, Australia, dengue diffused centripetally around the index case and by jump dispersal, creating new case clusters away from the index case (Vazquez-Prokopec et al. 2010). It was also found that new dengue infections spread at 14–32m per week and many cases clustered at 800m from the index case. These observations underscore the importance of efficient dengue surveillance systems in places with established dengue vector populations. Vector control in these examples consisted of focal control 100m around detected dengue cases using indoor residual insecticide spraying (IRS; lambda-cyhalothrin), source reduction, and larvicide (S-methoprene). Only when vector control coverage exceeded 60% of surrounding houses was there a significant impact on DENV containment. In situations where early detection of dengue cases is not possible, then the whole neighbourhood would need to be treated (Morrison et al. 1999).

7.1.1. Vector control recommendations for non-endemic areas

- Investigate each report of ATV-like disease and determine if it is imported or autochthonous.

- If an ATV case is detected, notify the residents and conduct a proactive search for more cases.

- Enhance entomological surveillance using traps for adult mosquitoes throughout the neighbourhood, and use GIS to keep tract of cases, mosquitoes, and control measures.

- Contain virus spread: initiate vector control in the entire neighbourhood, beginning with the areas with confirmed cases.

  o Conduct door-to-door visits to houses, lots, shops, industries, construction sites, schools, etc. Visits need to be coordinated to coincide with the presence of people in the premises. For example, household visits should be made at times when people are at home (after working hours, weekends, and holidays).

    ■ Provide educational materials and request the participation of residents in terms of eliminating water sources and reporting illness or symptoms.

    ■ Determine the main types of containers producing *Aedes* mosquitoes.

    ■ Establish if there is indoor production of mosquitoes in flowerpots, water basins, roof tanks, and underground cisterns or septic tanks.

    ■ Eliminate disposable containers.

    ■ Treat containers that cannot be removed with long-lasting larvicides and conduct residual insecticide spraying on container surfaces and adjacent mosquito resting sites.

  o Conduct general clean-up campaigns in private and public areas.

- o If allowed, conduct indoor/outdoor space spraying of insecticides targeting infected mosquitoes, and residual insecticides on surfaces where mosquitoes tend to land (dark areas indoors, and on containers and adjacent surfaces outdoors). Insecticides should be chosen carefully based on baseline studies of insecticide resistance.

- o Promote the use of repellents, proper clothing, bed nets for patients, and the use of screens in windows and doors.

7.2. Endemic/epidemic areas

ATV epidemics in endemic areas typically represent a collection of outbreaks, where the incidence is greater than would otherwise be expected at a particular time and place (e.g., >1% prevalence) (Newton and Reiter 1992). Thus, the main difficulty in controlling dengue epidemics is the extent of territory that would need to be covered to control mosquitoes in a short period of time. There is little evidence showing that dengue epidemics can be controlled (WHO 2009), but it is also difficult to evaluate the impact of vector control measures during epidemics because most resources are dedicated to fighting the outbreaks. A study conducted in Puerto Rico during a significant dengue outbreak concluded that, despite extensive efforts to control the epidemic being largely ineffective, future strategies should prioritize prevention rather than solely focusing on managing dengue outbreaks (Morens et al. 1986).

Extensive dengue vector control measures are favoured during epidemics since so many urban areas have their own ATV cases. Control measures are usually planned and monitored by a team of inter-agency officials including the state's departments of health, environment, public works, and education, as well as municipalities, armed force personnel, academic institutions, NGOs, etc. Control measures include spraying insecticide (adulticides/larvicides) with aircraft- or truck-mounted equipment, massive educational media campaigns (TV, radio, newspapers, talks, etc.), general clean-up efforts, participation from armed forces and volunteers to conduct door-to-door vector control, and improved case diagnosis and management through the training of physicians and nurses, and the improvement of hospital supplies (Morens et al. 1986, Pilger et al. 2010).

Another challenge is that the planning and implementation of control measures might take some time (Rigau-Perez and Gubler 1997), and epidemics are usually detected or declared during their phase of exponential increase in cases. Other problems related to controlling dengue epidemics are the ostensible lack of highly trained vector control personnel and insufficient budget allocation (Reiter and Gubler 1997).

Dengue epidemics can be anticipated several months in advance through the use of early warning systems. For instance, in Puerto Rico, an epidemic was predicted for 2010 when the number of suspected dengue cases exceeded a historical threshold (the seventy-fifth percentile of average weekly cases from 1986 to 2009) during epidemiological weeks four to five. The epidemic ultimately peaked during weeks thirty-two to thirty-four, providing a lead time of seven months for preparedness and response efforts (Fig. 7.1). The significant increase in dengue cases in January and February—when dengue cases in Puerto Rico have historically reached a seasonal minimum—implies that the conditions for the development of an epidemic were already happening at that time. Based on mathematical models, it has been shown that dengue epidemics take several months to develop, and that the magnitude of the epidemics depends on environmental conditions occurring very early in the process that cause high, initial virus reproduction rates (Focks and Barrera 2007). These observations suggest that to prevent dengue epidemics, vector control measures must start very early in the season during periods when environmental conditions would not seem to be conducive to dengue outbreaks, such as during the cooler and drier months of the boreal winter in Puerto Rico (Barrera 2015b). Furthermore, the carry-over of dengue transmission from one year to the next needs to be minimized.

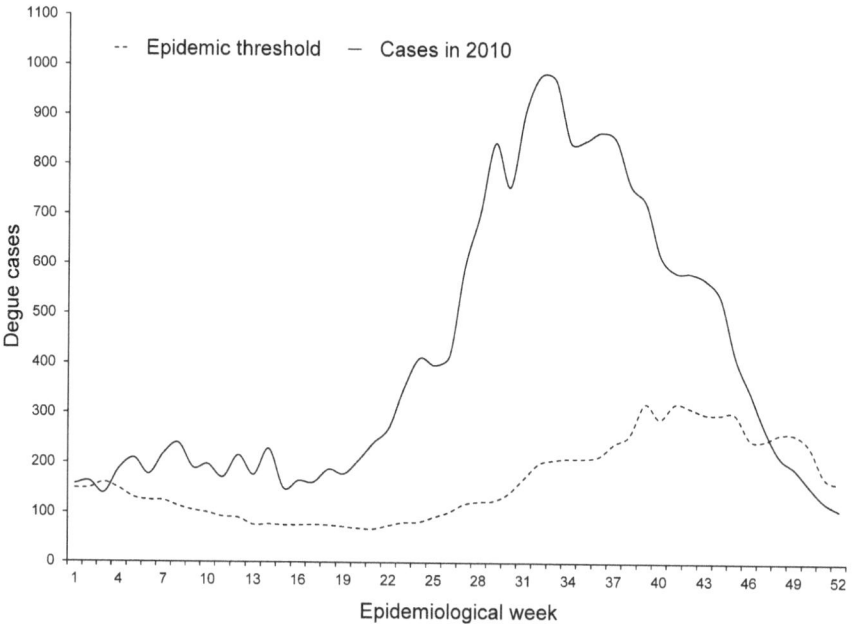

Fig. 7.1. A simple early warning system to predict the risk of an epidemic later in the year in Puerto Rico in 2010. The frequency of cases above the epidemic threshold for consecutive weeks early in the year predicted an impending epidemic.

Another factor that can contribute to the prevention of ATV epidemics is having appropriate spatial stratification of urban sectors based on historical disease incidence and persistence (Barrera et al. 2000). It has been shown that roughly the same neighbourhoods in Maracay city, Venezuela had the highest year-to-year dengue incidence, usually in the highly populated sectors with deficiencies in public services and elevated populations of *Ae. aegypti* (Barrera et al. 2002). It was also noted that approximately 70% of the cases were concentrated in 30% of the city's neighbourhoods. A study of the spatial-temporal patterns of historical dengue and Zika epidemics in the metropolitan area of San Juan, Puerto Rico (2010–2022) showed similar results, where 75% of cases were confirmed in 25% of the urban area (Barrera et al. 2024). Furthermore, most hot spots of epidemics of DENV (2010–2014 and 2015–2022) and ZIKV (2015–2017) had a high percentage of spatial overlap or spatial correlation, indicating the likely areas that will be the most impacted by future epidemics.

Because various dengue serotypes can co-circulate in dengue-endemic areas, there are always some serotypes that some people are susceptible to. Additionally, emerging ATVs such as chikungunya and Zika found human populations that had never experienced infections from these viruses, which led to explosive outbreaks in the Americas, including the US and territories. Knowledge of what urban sectors tend to have the highest dengue incidences can be used to conduct pre-emptive vector control well ahead of outbreaks, which usually present during the warmer and wetter part of the year (Barrera et al. 2011, Barrera et al. 2023).

7.2.1. Vector control recommendations for endemic/epidemic areas

7.2.1.1. Prevention of epidemics

- **Stratification/priority areas.** Pre-emptive vector control in neighbourhoods known to have been hot spots for ATV transmission should help to prevent the buildup and spread of epidemics. As explained earlier, dengue transmission is highly heterogeneous, with some neighbourhoods producing the bulk of dengue cases. Hot spots are areas where environmental conditions are appropriate (e.g., stable, and elevated mosquito populations) for sustained and elevated ATV transmission. Hot spots are expected to facilitate virus export to other neighbourhoods. Thus, effective vector control in hot spots should help to reduce dengue incidence in the hot spots as well as in other areas of the city. Information about the historical occurrence of ATVs at fine spatial scales can be used to elaborate risk stratification systems based on environmental, entomological, social, and epidemiological data (Siqueira-Junior et al. 2008, Porcasi et al. 2012, Vanlerberghe et al. 2017, Dzul-Manzanilla et al. 2021). Spatial patterns of abundance of vector populations within hotspots has been observed within neighbourhoods, and this information can help to make vector control more efficient by highlighting areas to concentrate efforts, allowing the vector control programme to cover more areas with the same personnel.

- **Timing vector control measures.** In order to maximize the benefits of vector control, it needs to be effective and sustained (Pontes et al. 2000). Thus, vector control should be applied preventively and maintained throughout the year. In cases when that is not possible, vector control interventions applied early in the season (e.g., before the rainy season) contribute to extended vector control and significant reductions in transmission (Chadee 2009). As discussed earlier, epidemics take time to develop and although it is not clear when the best time to apply preventive control measures is, it makes sense to intensify vector control when the density of mosquitoes is lower (e.g., dry, cool seasons), during inter-epidemic periods.

- In dengue-endemic areas, there are typically two patterns of serotype dynamics: a temporal succession of single dengue serotypes infecting human populations, often observed in more isolated urban areas; or the co-circulation of multiple dengue serotypes that alternate in frequency every few years. The introduction of a new dengue virus serotype or emerging ATV to an endemic area should prompt efforts to contain it, in much the same way as would be done in non-endemic areas. If these efforts are successful, then eventually these areas will cease to be (hyper-)endemic. This strategy would require and depend on enhanced virological surveillance targeting the new serotype and adequate vector control capabilities to contain the virus.

- **Vector control measures.** There are several challenges to preventing dengue epidemics. Some of the challenges include insufficiencies in the organization, trained personnel, and resources required to carry out widespread, sustained vector control. Additionally, there is lack of appropriate operational indicators of both virus transmission and vector abundance that would inform when preventive vector control has reduced the mosquito population below threshold transmission levels. One indicator that adequate vector control levels have been achieved is the lack of sustained, local virus transmission. However, passive ATV surveillance systems that are based on detecting disease cases lack the spatial resolution to detect active transmission at local scales, because most DENV and ZIKV infections do not result in overt disease (silent transmission). Moreover, vector indicators are primarily based on immature indices (e.g., HI <1%) that demand much labour and time, and in some cases underestimate the true vector prevalence (e.g., cryptic containers). Therefore, more research is needed to determine the mosquito density thresholds that prevent local ATV transmission, using simplified and reliable mosquito surveillance tools. If vector control programmes had well-defined mosquito density thresholds, they would be able to determine if vector control actions were effective, without needing to wait for epidemiological outcomes.

Dengue vectors' threshold levels based on indices of immature mosquito presence in household containers (House Index, Container Index, Breteau Index) that were defined to prevent urban yellow fever epidemics in the past (Connor and Monroe 1923, Brown 1977a) have been adopted to prevent dengue epidemics. However, indices based on the presence of immature stages are not well correlated with the abundance of adult mosquitoes that actually transmit ATVs (Focks 2003). Also, the frequent reports of dengue vectors using cryptic aquatic habitats to undergo immature development (Barrera 2016) imply that records based on surveys of immature mosquitoes may underestimate the true prevalence of dengue vectors in places with aquatic habitats that cannot be discovered using visual inspections. It is unlikely that universal mosquito density thresholds could be found because thresholds vary with ambient temperature, previous immunity level of the human population, rate of ATV introductions (Focks et al. 2007), and protective measures that modulate mosquito-human contact, such as use of window and door screens. In temperate areas, marked seasonal changes in temperature result in mosquito density thresholds based on ovitrap captures varying in time, as shown for *Ae. albopictus* in Italy (Carrieri et al. 2012). Ovitrap data showing more than three eggs of *Ae. aegypti* per ovitrap per day was associated with the occurrence of dengue haemorrhagic fever in Thailand (Mogi et al. 1990). The advent of efficient traps for capturing female dengue vectors currently allows better estimations of the abundance of mosquito populations in relation to their transmission potential, as well as accurate estimations of mosquito density thresholds preventing local outbreaks of ATVs. Several field studies conducted in Puerto Rico proposed that a density threshold of two or three gravid females of *Ae. aegypti* captured per AGO trap can prevent local ATVs outbreaks (Barrera et al. 2014a, 2014b, 2017, 2019a, 2019c). It was calculated that three gravid females of *Ae. aegypti* per AGO trap per week was equivalent to one female of this species per BG-Sentinel trap (with a black cover, without chemical attractants) per day, and to three eggs per day in ovitraps (Barrera et al. 2017). The latter result is similar to the threshold reported for Thailand (Mogi et al. 1990).

Sustained vector control could be achieved by a combination of source reduction, larvicide, residual insecticide spraying targeting mosquito resting sites, gravid traps, and enhanced vector surveillance to detect areas where vector control is not working properly. Vector surveillance should be conducted using tools that minimize labour, time, costs, and maximize spatial coverage. It also requires effective means of portraying and disseminating vector data in as close to real time as possible. For example, the Mexican Dengue Control Programme has shifted from conducting vector surveillance based on immature indices to a network of four ovitraps per city block and an electronic reporting GIS that keeps track of oviposition activity, vector control operations, and dengue cases (Hernandez-Avila et al. 2013). It is expected that this type of surveillance system will ultimately provide an indication of the threshold for ATV transmission in Mexico (e.g., minimum number of eggs per ovitrap). Thus, it is recommended that vector control programmes evaluate both vector surveillance efforts (comparing immature and adult indicators) and integrated vector control tools (measuring the degree of vector reduction and its protective effect).

7.2.1.2. Control of epidemics

To respond to epidemics, an emergency operations centre (epidemiologists, entomologists and vector control specialists, educators, media communicators, etc.) should be activated to jointly plan, work, and evaluate progress throughout the epidemic, involving other agencies such as: environmental agencies, public works, law enforcement, fire departments, and municipalities.

- Promote community education and participation:
  - o Use various media (TV, radio, social media apps, newspapers, door hangers, local organizations, lectures at clinics and schools, etc.) to demonstrate the life cycle of mosquitoes and their role in ATV transmission, how they can be controlled at home, disease symptoms, treatments, and recommendations.
  - o Provide instructions on how to manage each type of container according to their properties (rooting plants, bromeliads and tree holes, pails, paint trays, plastic pools, small and large discarded containers and appliances, plant trivets, water-storage containers, gutters and drains, septic tanks, water meters, ornamental fountains, bird baths, and pets' drinking pans).
  - o Report daily to the press about which neighbourhoods have dengue cases and what people can do to protect themselves and help to control transmission.
- Promote the use of bed nets for febrile or ill persons at unprotected homes and hospitals.
- Train physicians and nurses in dengue case diagnosis and treatment, and provide hospitals with needed resources.
- Enhance epidemiological and entomological surveillance.
- Orient vector control operations through real-time epidemiological and entomological indicators, and use GIS to map and report.
- Prioritize areas for vector control based on current and past arbovirus transmission (in the previous five to ten years).
- Vector control:
  - o Divide the target area (municipality) into smaller, operational control areas (e.g., census tracts, census blocks, neighbourhoods) where control measures will be applied

to all buildings and public areas within a few days, and repeat treatments as soon as possible.

o Conduct door-to-door inspections and mosquito control in an area-wide fashion (reach >90% coverage within a week).

o Train hired and volunteer personnel to identify and treat containers producing mosquitoes.

o Organize clean-up campaigns targeting disposable containers (source reduction) in buildings, public areas, etc.

o Combine indoor/outdoor spatial or residual spraying with source reduction and larvicide (including the residual spraying of container surfaces and adjacent mosquito resting areas, using effective insecticides).

o Select areas to evaluate the impact and frequency of control operations (neighbourhoods with enhanced entomological and epidemiological surveillance).

7.3. Key messages for the prevention of dengue

Key vector management messages for the prevention and control of dengue (CDC 2025c) should be based on specific behavioural objectives such as persuading residents to manage their household containers in ways that will reduce the production of mosquitoes, specifically targeting the most productive containers. We can learn how residents use and manipulate their containers in their environments to design the best prevention practices to avoid producing mosquitoes (Lloyd 2003). Consequently, a health communications team can develop messages for the specific behavioural objective and collaborate with media partners to decide what educational materials and media would be the most appropriate. The Centers for Disease Control and Prevention (CDC) provide several fact sheets and posters in English and Spanish on the mosquito life cycle, how to get rid of mosquitoes, disease symptoms, etc., that can be freely used and adapted (CDC 2024a).

7.3.1. Key messages for primary prevention

- **Dengue-endemic areas.** Educational materials and messages should be behaviourally-focused and disseminated before the beginning of the dengue season and during outbreaks to: (1) promote specific prevention practices based on the most productive and common containers producing mosquitoes, addressed to the target audience most likely to be responsible for these containers (e.g., the head of household, for water cisterns and septic tanks); (2) suggest personal protection measures for parents, youth, adults, and pregnant women, such as appropriate clothing; and (3) reduce exposure to mosquito bites at home through indoor insecticide, window and door screens, bed nets, and air conditioning.

- **Non dengue-endemic areas.** Risk communications and prevention messages should be disseminated to raise awareness of the potential occurrence of outbreaks, promote behavioural changes to avoid virus transmission, and inform about the response plan that would be implemented. Prevention messages need to address household elimination or control of water-holding containers as well as personal precautions to avoid mosquito bites.

- **Travellers.** Dengue prevention messages for travellers should address the importance of seeking pre-travel consultation before traveling to the tropics and subtropics, to receive advice about how to avoid mosquito bites (e.g., the use of repellents and appropriate clothing to wear, sleeping in rooms with screens and air conditioning, using mosquito nets, and applying domestic indoor insecticides). Travellers should be informed about ATVs, disease symptoms, and warning signs for severe manifestations, and urged to seek medical care if they develop dengue-like symptoms during travel or within two weeks of returning from travel.

7.3.2. Key messages for secondary prevention

The spread of dengue to other family members should be prevented. Mosquitoes that bite a sick family member can go on to infect others. Messages for caregivers should explain that the patient needs to rest under a bed net or use insect repellent while feverish to prevent other family members from being infected. All the mosquitoes in the house must be killed and all containers with water in and around yards must be emptied. If possible, caregivers should place screens on windows and doors or use air conditioning to prevent mosquitoes from entering the house.

8. Personal Protection Against Mosquito Bites and Recommendations for Improving Surveillance and Control

Reducing mosquito-human contact is critical for preventing dengue transmission. Effective personal protection methods include using window and door screens, bed nets (especially for febrile patients), topical repellents, area repellents, and insecticide-treated clothing. While bed nets may be less effective during the day when *Aedes* mosquitoes are active, they are essential for isolating infected individuals. Recommended repellents include DEET, picaridin, oil of lemon eucalyptus, IR3535, and para-menthane-diol, whose effectiveness is influenced by concentration and environmental factors. Area repellents, primarily pyrethroids, can create mosquito-free zones, while permethrin-treated clothing offers extended protection. Product effectiveness depends on proper use and local mosquito susceptibility.

This chapter also highlights key strategies to enhance dengue vector surveillance and control in the US and territories. It calls for improved monitoring systems using GIS, novel mosquito traps, and routine insecticide resistance assessments. Emphasis is placed on targeting non-endemic areas and fostering collaboration and data sharing. Integrated vector management (IVM), community engagement, and ongoing research into control agents are essential for effective intervention. Finally, this chapter stresses the importance of resistance management, pre-emptive control in high-risk areas, and capacity building for vector control personnel to ensure long-term, sustainable mosquito and disease control efforts.

     https://doi.org/10.11647/OBP.0472.08

Reducing mosquito-human contact is essential for dengue prevention and control because it decreases the possibility of humans being bitten by infected mosquitoes and reduces feeding opportunities for mosquitoes. Protection against mosquito bites can be achieved by using screens in windows and doors, bed nets, topic and area repellents, and approved insecticide-impregnated clothing.

It has been shown that having screens in windows and doors is a protective factor against dengue infections (Waterman et al. 1985). The use of bed nets to prevent dengue infections is controversial because most people are not in bed during the day when dengue vectors bite. However, in dengue-endemic areas, everybody who is bed-ridden with a high fever should use a bed net. Patients who have been diagnosed with dengue should stay under a bed net in unprotected homes or in hospital to avoid infecting mosquitoes. If bed nets are impregnated with residual insecticide, there is an opportunity to reduce the number of mosquitoes in the home and protect others, but the type of insecticide needs to be one which local dengue vectors are susceptible to.

The following topic repellents are commonly found in stores and recommended, as they provide reasonably long-lasting protection (CDC 2024b, EPA 2025b):

- **DEET** (chemical name: N,N-diethyl-m-toluamide or N,N-diethyl-3-methyl-benzamide). This repellent is effective at repelling mosquitoes, sand flies, biting midges, stable flies, black flies, fleas, ticks, and chiggers (Xue et al. 2007).

- **Icaridin (Picaridin)** (KBR 3023; chemical name: 2-(2-hydroxyethyl)-1-piperidinecarboxylic acid 1-methylpropyl ester). This repellent is used against mosquitoes and ticks.

- **Oil of lemon eucalyptus** (OLE) (chemical name: para-menthane-3,8-diol; the synthesized version of OLE). This repellent is used against mosquitoes and ticks.

- **IR3535** (chemical name: 3-[N-butyl-N-acetyl]-aminopropionic acid, ethyl ester). This repellent is used against mosquitoes and ticks.

- **Para-menthane-diol** (PMD). This product, made from extracts of eucalyptus plants, is used against mosquitoes.

The duration of protection is a function of product concentration but is also affected by ambient temperature, level of activity, amount of perspiration, exposure to water, abrasive removal, and other factors. Regardless of what product is used, repellent application should be made according to label instructions.

Chemical space-area repellents are designed to protect people from being reached and bitten by mosquitoes within a given area (room, picnic table, etc.). Most area repellent chemicals are pyrethroids. They can be dispensed using vaporization products (coils, electric heating impregnated paper mats, and candles). The pyrethroids metofluthrin and transfluthrin are highly volatile and do not need vaporizers. They are usually delivered as impregnated materials and hung in rooms (Strickman 2007).

Clothes can be impregnated with 0.05% permethrin for protection against mosquitoes, ticks, and other biting insects. Permethrin-treated clothing can be purchased in the US. Permethrin-treated materials retain repellence after repeated laundering but should be re-treated, as described on the product label, to provide continued protection. As with any insecticide, the effectiveness of permethrin may vary depending on the susceptibility of local mosquito strains.

8.1. Surveillance and monitoring

- **Enhanced surveillance systems.** There is a clear need for improved surveillance systems to monitor and report the distribution of dengue vectors across geographical regions in the US and territories. This includes establishing routine monitoring in areas previously considered low risk to detect any emerging threats early. GIS should be utilized to track cases and mosquito populations in real time.

- **Focus on non-endemic areas.** Special attention should be given to non-endemic areas where vectors have been introduced. Strategies should be developed to prevent the establishment of persistent populations and to mitigate the risk of local transmission.

- **Development of novel trapping technologies.** Investing in the development and deployment of innovative trapping technologies can improve the capture of adult mosquitoes. This includes refining existing traps and exploring new designs that enhance attraction and retention of target species.

- **Regular monitoring of insecticide resistance.** Establishing routine monitoring programmes to assess the levels of insecticide resistance in dengue vector populations is essential. This should include both laboratory assays and field evaluations of commercial products to track changes over time and across geographical regions.

- **Collaboration and data sharing.** Encouraging collaboration among public health agencies, researchers, and vector control programmes can facilitate data sharing and enhance understanding of resistance dynamics. This collaboration can lead to more effective and coordinated resistance management efforts.

8.2. Vector control strategies

- **Integrated vector management (IVM).** Enhance IVM programmes that combine multiple control strategies— including chemical, biological, and environmental methods— to target all life stages of dengue vectors. Foster collaboration among various governmental and non-governmental organizations to coordinate vector control efforts, share resources, and implement comprehensive strategies.

- **Sustained community engagement.** Maintain ongoing community education and engagement efforts, even outside of outbreak periods, to ensure continued awareness and participation in dengue prevention. Encourage community involvement in vector control efforts, such as clean-up campaigns and source reduction initiatives, fostering a sense of ownership and responsibility.

- **Research on control agents.** Continued research is needed to identify and develop effective control agents, including novel insecticides, and biological control methods. Understanding the long-term impacts, costs, and sustainability of these approaches is critical for their successful implementation.

- **Evaluation of control strategies.** Establishing clear metrics for evaluating the effectiveness of vector control interventions is necessary. Longitudinal studies should be conducted to assess the impact of various control measures on mosquito populations and disease transmission over time. Conduct research to establish mosquito density thresholds that correlate with the risk of dengue transmission, allowing for timely interventions based on surveillance data.

- **Pre-emptive vector control.** Conduct pre-emptive vector control in historically high-risk neighbourhoods to prevent the buildup of mosquito populations.

- **Long-term monitoring.** Conduct continuous research on the genetic and ecological dynamics of *Aedes* species to inform future control strategies.

- **Development of resistance management strategies.** Implementing comprehensive resistance management strategies that incorporate multiple approaches can help to delay the development of resistance. This includes rotating insecticides with different modes of action, using mixtures of insecticides, and integrating non-chemical control methods.

- **Capacity building for vector control personnel.** Invest in training programmes for vector control personnel to ensure they are equipped with the necessary skills and knowledge to implement effective control measures.

References

Acevedo V, Amador M, Barrera R. Improving the safety and acceptability of Autocidal Gravid Ovitraps (AGO traps). *J Am Mosq Control Assoc.* 2021;37(2):61–7, https://doi.org/10.2987/21-6996.1

Adams B, Boots M. How important is vertical transmission in mosquitoes for the persistence of dengue? Insights from a mathematical model. *Epidemics.* 2010;2:1–10, https://doi.org/10.1016/j.epidem.2010.01.001

Adams LE, Martin SW, Lindsey NP, Lehman JA, Rivera A, Kolsin J, Landry K, Staples JE, Sharp TM, Paz-Bailey G, Fischer M. Epidemiology of dengue, chikungunya, and Zika virus disease in U.S. states and territories, 2017. *Am J Trop Med Hyg.* 2019;101(4):884–90, https://doi.org/10.4269/ajtmh.19-0309

Agudelo-Silva F, Spielman A. Paradoxical effects of simulated larviciding on production of adult mosquitoes. *Am J Trop Med Hyg.* 1984;33(6):1267–1269, https://doi.org/10.4269/ajtmh.1984.33.1267

Ahmed M, Pollak NM, Hugo LE, van den Hurk AF, Hobson-Peters J, Macdonald J. Rapid molecular assays for the detection of the four dengue viruses in infected mosquitoes. *Gates Open Res.* 2022;6:81, https://doi.org/10.12688/gatesopenres.13534.2

Alexander N, Lenhart AE, Romero-Vivas CME, Barbazan P, Morrison AC, Barrera R, et al. Sample sizes for identifying the key types of container occupied by dengue-vector pupae: the use of entropy in analyses of compositional data. *Ann Trop Med Parasitol.* 2006;100:S5–16, https://doi.org/10.1179/136485906X105471

Ali A, Nayar JK, Xue R. Comparative toxicity of selected larvicides and insect growth regulators to a Florida laboratory population of *Aedes albopictus. J Am Mosq Control Assoc.* 1995;11(1):72–6

Alphey L, McKemey A, Nimmo D, Neira Oviedo M, Lacroix R, Matzen K, et al. Genetic control of *Aedes* mosquitoes. *Pathog Glob Health.* 2013;107(4):170–9, https://doi.org/10.1179/2047773213Y.0000000095

Amarakoon D, Chen A, Rawlins S, Chadee DD, Taylor M, Stennett R. Dengue epidemics in the Caribbean-temperature indices to gauge the potential for onset of dengue. *Mitig Adapt Strateg Glob Chang.* 2008;13(4):341–57, https://doi.org/10.1007/s11027-007-9114-5

Anderson AL, Apperson CS, Knake R. Effectiveness of mist-blower applications of malathion and permethrin to foliage as barrier sprays for salt marsh mosquitoes. *J Am Mosq Control Assoc.* 1991;7(1):116–7.

Anez G, Rios M. Dengue in the United States of America: a worsening scenario? *Biomed Res Int.* 2013;2013, https://doi.org/10.1155/2013/678645

Anyamba A, Chretien JP, Britch SC, Soebiyanto RP, Small JL, Jepsen R, Forshey BM, Sanchez JL, Smith RD, Harris R, Tucker CJ. Global disease outbreaks associated with the 2015-2016 El Niño event. *Sci Rep.* 2019;9(1):1930, https://doi.org/10.1038/s41598-018-38034-z

Arima Y, Edelstein ZR, Hana HK, Matsui T. Epidemiologic update on the dengue situation in the Western Pacific Region, 2011. *Western Pac Surveill Response.* 2013;4(2):47–54, https://doi.org/10.5365/WPSAR.2012.3.4.019

Asish PR, Dasgupta S, Rachel G, Bagepally BS, Girish Kumar CP. Global prevalence of asymptomatic dengue infections - a systematic review and meta-analysis. *Int J Infect Dis.* 2023;134:292–8, https://doi.org/10.1016/j.ijid.2023.07.010

Aubry M, Teissier A, Roche C, Richard V, Yan AS, Zisou K, et al. Chikungunya outbreak, French Polynesia, 2014. *Emerg Infect Dis.* 2015;21(4):724–6, https://doi.org/10.3201/eid2104.141741

Azil AH, Li M, R. WC. Dengue vector surveillance programmes: a review of methodological diversity in some endemic and epidemic countries. *Asia Pac J Public Health.* 2011;23:827–42, https://doi.org/10.1177/1010539511426595

Azil AH, Long SA, Ritchie SA, Williams CR. The development of predictive tools for pre-emptive dengue vector control: a study of *Aedes aegypti* abundance and meteorological variables in North Queensland, Australia. *Trop Med Int Health.* 2010;15(10):1190–7, https://doi.org/10.1111/j.1365-3156.2010.02592.x

Bailey SF, Bohart RM. A mosquito survey and control programme in Guam. *J Econ Entomol.* 1953;45(6):947–52.

Ball TS, Ritchie SR. Evaluation of BG-sentinel trap trapping efficacy for *Aedes aegypti* (Diptera: Culicidae) in a visually competitive environment. *J Med Entomol.* 2010;47(4):657–63, https://doi.org/10.1603/me09242

Bangs MJ, Pudiantari R, Gionar YR. Persistence of dengue virus RNA in dried *Aedes aegypti* (Diptera : Culicidae) exposed to natural tropical conditions. *J Med Entomol.* 2007;44(1):163–7, https://doi.org/10.1603/0022-2585(2007)44[163:podvri]2.0.co;2

Bargielowski IE, Lounibos LP. Satyrization and satyrization-resistance in competitive displacements of invasive mosquito species. *Insect Sci.* 2015;23(2):162–74, https://doi.org/10.1111/1744-7917.12291

Barrera R. Competition and resistance to starvation in larvae of container-inhabiting *Aedes* mosquitoes. *Ecol. Entomol.* 1996;21(2):117–27, https://doi.org/10.1111/j.1365-2311.1996.tb01178.x

Barrera R. Simplified pupal surveys of *Aedes aegypti* (L.) for entomologic surveillance and dengue control. *Am J Trop Med Hyg.* 2009;81(1):100–7, https://doi.org/10.4269/ajtmh.2009.81.100

Barrera R. Dinámica del dengue y *Aedes aegypti* in Puerto Rico. *Rev Biomédica.* 2010;21:179–95.

Barrera R. Spatial stability of adult *Aedes aegypti* populations. *Am J Trop Med Hyg.* 2011;85(6):1087–92, https://doi.org/10.4269/ajtmh.2011.11-0381

Barrera R. [Dengue and chikungunya vector control: Is it necessary to re-examine present strategies?]. *Biomédica.* 2015a;35(3):297–9, https://doi.org/10.7705/biomedica.v35i3

Barrera R. Considerations for disrupting dengue virus transmission: ecology of *Aedes aegypti* and current (non genetic) methods of control. In: Adelman ZN, editor. Genetic Control of Malaria and Dengue (Oxford: Academic Press, 2015b, pp. 103–24).

Barrera R. Recomendaciones para el monitoreo de *Aedes aegypti. Biomédica.* 2016;36(3):454–462, https://doi.org/10.7705/biomedica.v36i3.2892

Barrera R. New tools for *Aedes* control: mass trapping. *Curr Opin Insect Sci.* 2022;52:100942, https://doi.org/10.1016/j.cois.2022.100942

Barrera R, Acevedo V, Amador M, Marzan M, Adams LE, Paz-Bailey G. El Niño Southern Oscillation (ENSO) effects on local weather, arboviral diseases, and dynamics of managed and unmanaged populations of *Aedes aegypti* (Diptera: Culicidae) in Puerto Rico. *J Med Entomol.* 2023;60(4):796–807, https://doi.org/10.1093/jme/tjad053

Barrera R, Acevedo V, Felix GE, Hemme RR, Vazquez J, Munoz JL, et al. Impact of Autocidal Gravid Ovitraps on chikungunya virus incidence in *Aedes aegypti* (Diptera: Culicidae) in areas with and without traps. *J Med Entomol.* 2017;54(2):387–95, https://doi.org/10.1093/jme/tjw187

Barrera R, Amador M, Acevedo V, Beltran M, Muñoz JL. A comparison of mosquito densities, weather and infection rates of *Aedes aegypti* during the first epidemics of chikungunya (2014) and Zika (2016) in areas with and without vector control in Puerto Rico. *Med Vet Entomol.* 2019a;33(1):68–77, https://doi.org/10.1111/mve.12338

Barrera R, Amador M, Acevedo V, Caban B, Felix G, Mackay A. Use of the CDC Autocidal Gravid Ovitrap to control and prevent outbreaks of *Aedes aegypti* (Diptera: Culicidae). *J Med Entomol.* 2014;51(1):145–54, https://doi.org/10.1603/me13096

Barrera R, Amador M, Acevedo V, Hemme RR, Felix G. Sustained, area-wide control of *Aedes aegypti* using CDC autocidal gravid ovitraps. *Am J Trop Med Hyg*. 2014a;91(6):1269–76, https://doi.org/10.4269/ajtmh.14-0426

Barrera R, Amador M, Clark GG. The use of household bleach to control *Aedes aegypti*. *J Am Mosq Control Assoc*. 2004;20(4):444–8.

Barrera R, Amador M, Clark GG. Sample-size requirements for developing strategies, based on the pupal/demographic survey, for the targeted control of dengue. *Ann Trop Med Parasitol*. 2006a;100(suppl 1):S33–S43, https://doi.org/10.1179/136485906X105499

Barrera R, Amador M, Clark GG. Use of the pupal survey technique for measuring *Aedes aegypti* (Diptera: Culicidae) productivity in Puerto Rico. *Am J Trop Med Hyg*. 2006b;74(2):290–302, https://doi.org/10.4269/ajtmh.2006.74.290

Barrera R, Amador M, Diaz A, Smith J, Munoz-Jordan JL, Rosario Y. Unusual productivity of *Aedes aegypti* in septic tanks and its implications for dengue control. *Med Vet Entomol*. 2008;22(1):62–9, https://doi.org/10.1111/j.1365-2915.2008.00720.x

Barrera R, Amador M, MacKay AJ. Population dynamics of *Aedes aegypti* and dengue as influenced by weather and human behavior in San Juan, Puerto Rico. *PLoS Negl Trop Dis*. 2011;5(12):e1378, https://doi.org/10.1371/journal.pntd.0001378

Barrera R, Amador M, Munoz J, Acevedo V. Integrated vector control of *Aedes aegypti* mosquitoes around target houses. *Parasit Vectors*. 2018;11(1):88, https://doi.org/10.1186/s13071-017-2596-4

Barrera R, Avila J, Gonzalez-tellez S. Unreliable supply of potable water and elevated *Aedes aegypti* larval indexes - a causal relationship. *J Am Mosq Control Assoc*. 1993;9(2):189–95.

Barrera R, Avila J, Navarro JC. Population dynamics of *Aedes aegypti* (L.) in urban areas with deficient supply of potable water. *Acta Biol Venez*. 1996;16:23–35.

Barrera R, Bingham AM, Hassan HK, Amador M, Mackay AJ, Unnasch TR. Vertebrate hosts of *Aedes aegypti* and *Aedes mediovittatus* (Diptera: Culicidae) in rural Puerto Rico. *J Med Entomol*. 2012;49(4):917–21, https://doi.org/10.1603/me12046

Barrera R, Delgado N, Jimenez M, Valero S. Eco-epidemiological factors associated with hyperendemic dengue hemorrhagic fever in Maracay City, Venezuela. *Dengue Bull*. 2002;26:84–95.

Barrera R, Delgado N, Jimenez M, Villalobos I, Romero I. [Stratification of a hyperendemic city in hemorrhagic dengue]. *Rev Panam Salud Publica*. 2000;8(4):225–33, https://doi.org/10.1590/s1020-49892000000900001

Barrera R, Felix G, Acevedo V, Amador M, Rodriguez D, Rivera L, Gonzalez O, Nazario N, Ortiz M, Muñoz-Jordan JL, Waterman SH. Impacts of Hurricanes Irma and Maria on *Aedes aegypti* populations, aquatic habitats, and mosquito infections with dengue, chikungunya, and Zika viruses in Puerto Rico. *Am J Trop Med Hyg*. 2019b;100(6):1413–1420, https://doi.org/10.4269/ajtmh.19-0015

Barrera R, Harris A, Hemme RR, Felix G, Nazario N, Muñoz-Jordan JL, et al. Citywide control of *Aedes aegypti* (Diptera: Culicidae) during the 2016 Zika epidemic by integrating community awareness, education, source reduction, larvicides, and mass mosquito trapping. *J Med Entomol*. 2019c;56(4):1033–46, https://doi.org/10.1093/jme/tjz009

Barrera R, Mackay AJ, Amador M. A novel autocidal ovitrap for the surveillance and control of *Aedes aegypti*. *J Am Mosq Control Assoc*. 2013a;29:293–6, https://doi.org/10.2987/13-6345R.1

Barrera R, Mackay AJ, Amador M. An improved trap to capture adult container-inhabiting mosquitoes. *J Am Mosq Control Assoc*. 2013b;29:358–68, https://doi.org/10.2987/13-6343.1

Barrera R, Medialdea V. Development time and resistance to starvation of mosquito larvae. *J Nat Hist*. 1996;30:447–58, https://doi.org/10.1080/00222939600770231

Barrera R, Navarro JC, Mora JD, Dominguez D, Gonzalez J. Public service deficiencies and *Aedes aegypti* breeding sites in Venezuela. *Bull Pan Am Health Organ*. 1995;29(3):193–205.

Barrera R, Ruiz J, Adams LE, Marzan-Rodriguez M, Paz-Bailey G. Historical hot spots of dengue and Zika viruses to guide targeted vector control in San Juan, Puerto Rico (2010-2022). *Am J Trop Med Hyg*. 2024;110(4):731–737, https://doi.org/10.4269/ajtmh.23-0627

Bellini R, Medici A, Puggioli A, Balestrino F, Carrieri M. Pilot field trials with *Aedes albopictus* irradiated sterile males in Italian urban areas. *J Med Entomol*. 2013;50(2):317–25, https://doi.org/10.1603/me12048

Bennett JK, Hickman AD, Kline MA, McGinnis MW, Weissmann MJ, Bennett JK, et al. New state record for the Asian tiger mosquito, *Aedes albopictus* (Skuse). *J Am Mosq Control Assoc*. 2005;21(4):341–3, https://doi.org/10.2987/8756-971X(2006)21[341:NSRFTA]2.0.CO;2

Bhalala H, Arias JR. The Zumba mosquito trap and BG-Sentinel trap: novel surveillance tools for host-seeking mosquitoes. *J Am Mosq Control Assoc*. 2009;25(2):134–9, https://doi.org/10.2987/08-5821.1

Bibbs CS, Anderson CS, Smith ML, Xue R-D. Direct and indirect efficacy of truck-mounted applications of s-methoprene against *Aedes albopictus* (Diptera: Culicidae). *Int J Pest Manag*. 2018;64(1):19–26, https://doi.org/10.1080/09670874.2017.1293308

Black WCI, Rai KS, Turco BJ, Arroyo DC. Laboratory study of competition between Unites States strains of *Aedes albopictus* and *Aedes aegypti* (Diptera: Culicidae). *J Med Entomol*. 1989;26(4):260–71, https://doi.org/10.1093/jmedent/26.4.260

Bouri N, Sell TK, Franco C, Adalja AA, Henderson DA, Hynes NA. Return of epidemic dengue in the United States: implications for the public health practitioner. *Public Health Rep*. 2012;127(3):259–66, https://doi.org/10.1177/003335491212700305

Boyce R, Lenhart A, Kroeger A, Velayudhan R, Roberts B, Horstick O. *Bacillus thuringiensis israelensis* (Bti) for the control of dengue vectors: systematic literature review. *Trop Med Int Health*. 2013;18(5):564–77, https://doi.org/10.1111/tmi.12087

Braga IA, Mello CB, Montella IR, Lima JBP, Junior AJM, Medeiros PFV, et al. Effectiveness of methoprene, an insect growth regulator, against temephos-resistant *Aedes aegypti* populations from different Brazilian localities, under laboratory conditions. *J Med Entomol*. 2005;42(5):830–7, https://doi.org/10.1093/jmedent/42.5.830

Brathwaite O, Martin JLS, Montoya HR, Zambrano B, Dayan GH. The history of dengue outbreaks in the Americas. *Am J Trop Med Hyg*. 2011;1:94, https://doi.org/10.4269/ajtmh.2012.11-0770

Brogdon WG, McAllister JC. Simplification of adult mosquito bioassays through use of time-mortality determinations in glass bottles. *J Am Mosq Control Assoc*. 1998;14(2):159–64.

Brown A. *Yellow Fever, Dengue and Dengue Haemorrhagic Fever. A World Geography of Human Diseases* (London: Academic Press, 1977a, pp. 271–316).

Brown AWA. *World Wide Surveillance of Aedes aegypti* (Visalia, CA: CMCA Press, 1977b, pp. 271–316).

Burke RL, Barrera R, Kluchinsky T, Lewis M, Claborn DM. Examination of a miniaturized funnel trap for *Aedes aegypti* (Diptera: Culicidae) larval sampling. *J Med Entomol*. 2010;47(6):1231–4, https://doi.org/10.1603/me10112

Burkhalter KL, Lindsay R, Anderson R, Dibernardo A, Fong W, Nasci RS. Evaluation of commercial assays for detecting West Nile virus antigen. *J Am Mosq Control Assoc*. 2006;22(1):64–9, https://doi.org/10.2987/8756-971X(2006)22[64:EOCAFD]2.0.CO;2

Burkhalter KL, Savage HM. Detection of Zika Virus in desiccated mosquitoes by real-time reverse transcription PCR and plaque assay. *Emerg Infect Dis*. 2017;23(4):680–1, https://doi.org/10.3201/eid2304.161772

Burkot TR, Handzel T, Schmaedick MA, Tufa J, Roberts JM, Graves PM. Productivity of natural and artificial containers for *Aedes polynesiensis* and *Aedes aegypti* in four American Samoan villages. *Med Vet Entomol.* 2007;21(1):22–9, https://doi.org/10.1111/j.1365-2915.2007.00667.x

Burkot TR, Melrose WD, Durrheim DN, Speare R, Ichimori K. *Impact of Mass Drug Administration on Aedes-Transmitted Filariasis in the Pacific* (Geneva, Switzerland: TDR/WHO, 2005).

Camargo S. History of *Aedes aegypti* eradication in the Americas. *Bull WHO.* 1967;36(4):602-603).

Carrieri M, Angelini P, Venturelli C, Maccagnani B, Bellini R. *Aedes albopictus* (Diptera: Culicidae) Population size survey in the 2007 chikungunya outbreak area in Italy. II: estimating epidemic thresholds. *J Med Entomol.* 2012;49(2):388–99, https://doi.org/10.1603/ME10259

Carter HR. *Yellow Fever. An Epidemiologic and Historical Study of Its Place of Origin* (Baltimore, MD: Williams & Wilkins Co, 1931), https://doi.org/10.4269/ajtmh.2000.62.378

Casas-Martinez M, Orozco-Bonilla A, Munoz-Reyes M, Ulloa-Garcia A, Bond JG, Valle-Mora J, et al. A new tent trap for monitoring the daily activity of *Aedes aegypti* and *Aedes albopictus. J Vector Ecol.* 2013;38(2):277–88, https://doi.org/10.1111/j.1948-7134.2013.12041.x

CDC. *CONUS Manual for Evaluating Insecticide Resistance in Mosquitoes Using the CDC Bottle Bioassay Kit.* (Centers for Disease Control and Prevention, 2020), https://www.cdc.gov/mosquitoes/pdfs/conus-508.pdf

CDC. Dengue. Life cycle of *Aedes* mosquitoes [Internet]. CDC;2024a [cited 19 May 2025], https://www.cdc.gov/mosquitoes/about/life-cycle-of-Aedes-mosquitoes.html#cdc_generic_section_3-fact-sheets

CDC. Dengue. Preventing mosquito bites [Internet]. CDC;2024b [cited 19 May 2025], https://www.cdc.gov/mosquitoes/prevention/index.html#:~:text=Use%20Environmental%20Protection%20Agency%20.

CDC Dengue. Current year data (2025) [Internet]. CDC;2025a [cited 19 May 2025], https://www.cdc.gov/dengue/data-research/facts-stats/current-data.html

CDC Dengue. Historic data (2010-2024) [Internet]. CDC;2025b [cited 19 May 2025], https://www.cdc.gov/dengue/data-research/facts-stats/historic-data.html

CDC Dengue. Preventing dengue [Internet]. CDC;2025c [cited 19 May 2025], https://www.cdc.gov/dengue/prevention/index.html

Chadee DD. Impact of pre-seasonal focal treatment on population densities of the mosquito *Aedes aegypti* in Trinidad, West Indies: A preliminary study. *Acta Trop.* 2009;109(3):236–40, https://doi.org/10.1016/j.actatropica.2008.12.001

Chadee DD, Ritchie SA. Oviposition behaviour and parity rates of *Aedes aegypti* collected in sticky traps in Trinidad, West Indies. *Acta Trop.* 2010;116(3):212–6, https://doi.org/10.1016/j.actatropica.2010.08.008

Challet GL. Elements of a vector control programme. *J Am Mosq Control Assoc.* 1991;7(1):103–6.

Chambers EW, McClintock SK, Avery MF, King JD, Bradley MH, Schmaedick MA, et al. Xenomonitoring of *Wuchereria bancrofti* and *Dirofilaria immitis* infections in mosquitoes from American Samoa: trapping considerations and a comparison of Polymerase chain reaction assays with dissection. *Am J Trop Med Hyg.* 2009;80(5):774–81, https://doi.org/10.4269/ajtmh.2009.80.774

Chan KL, Ho BC, Chan YC. *Aedes aegypti* (L.) and *Aedes albopictus* (Skuse) in Singapore City. 2. Larval habitats. *Bull WHO.* 1971;44:629–33.

Chan M, Johansson MA. The Incubation periods of dengue viruses. *PLoS One.* 2012;7(11), https://doi.org/10.1371/journal.pone.0050972

Chandler AC. Factors influencing the uneven distribution of *Aedes aegypti* in Texas cities. *Am J Trop Med Hyg.* 1945;25(2):145–9, https://doi.org/10.4269/ajtmh.1945.s1-25.145

Chandra G, Bhattacharjee I, Chatterjee SN, Ghosh A. Mosquito control by larvivorous fish. *Indian J Med Res.* 2008;127(1):13–27.

Chen CF, Shu PY, Teng HJ, Su CL, Wu JW, Wang JH, et al. Screening of dengue virus in field-caught *Aedes aegypti* and *Aedes albopictus* (Diptera: Culicidae) by one-step SYBR green-based reverse transcriptase-polymerase chain reaction assay during 2004-2007 in Southern Taiwan. *Vector Borne Zoonotic Dis.* 2010;10(10):1017–25, https://doi.org/10.1089/vbz.2008.0069

Chow VTK, Chan YC, Yong R, Lee KM, Lim LK, Chung YK, et al. Monitoring of dengue viruses in field-caught *Aedes aegypti* and *Aedes albopictus* mosquitoes by a type-specific Polymerase chain reaction and Cycle Sequencing. *Am J Trop Med Hyg.* 1998;58(5):578–86, https://doi.org/10.4269/ajtmh.1998.58.578

Christophers SR. *Aedes aegypti, the Yellow Fever Mosquito: Its Life History, Bionomics, and Structure* (London: Cambridge University Press, 1960).

Chung YK, Pang FY. Dengue virus infection rate in field populations of female *Aedes aegypti* and *Aedes albopictus* in Singapore. *Trop Med Int Health.* 2002;7(4):322–30, https://doi.org/10.1046/j.1365-3156.2002.00873.x

Cilek JE. Application of insecticides to vegetation as barriers against host-seeking mosquitoes. *J Am Mosq Control Assoc.* 2008;24(1):172–6, https://doi.org/10.2987/8756-971X(2008)24[172:AOITVA]2.0.CO;2

Clark G. Dengue and dengue hemorrhagic fever in Northern Mexico and South Texas: do they really respect the border? *Am J Trop Med Hyg.* 2008;78:361–2, https://doi.org/10.4269/ajtmh.2008.78.361

Clark GG, Seda H, Gubler DJ. Use of the "CDC backpack aspirator" for surveillance of *Aedes aegypti* in San Juan, Puerto Rico. *J Am Mosq Control Assoc*. 1994;10(1):119–24.

Connor M, Monroe W. Stegomyia indices and their value in yellow fever control. *Am J Trop Med Hyg*. 1923;3(1):9–19.

Corbel V, Kont MD, Ahumada ML, Andréo L, Bayili B, Bayili K, et al. A new WHO bottle bioassay method to assess the susceptibility of mosquito vectors to public health insecticides: results from a WHO-coordinated multi-centre study. *Parasit Vectors*. 2023;16(1):21, https://doi.org/10.1186/s13071-022-05554-7

Costero A, Attardo GM, Scott TW, Edman JD. An experimental study on the detection of fructose in *Aedes aegypti*. *J Am Mosq Control Assoc*. 1998;14(3):234–42.

Cox J, Grillet ME, Ramos OM, Amador M, Barrera R. Habitat segregation of dengue vectors along an urban environmental gradient. *Am J Trop Med Hyg*. 2007;76(5):820–6, https://doi.org/10.4269/ajtmh.2007.76.820

Crawford JE, Clarke DW, Criswell V, Desnoyer M, Cornel D, Deegan B, et al. Efficient production of male *Wolbachia*-infected *Aedes aegypti* mosquitoes enables large-scale suppression of wild populations. *Nat Biotechnol*. 2020;38(4):482–92, https://doi.org/10.1038/s41587-020-0471-x

Degallier N, Servain J, Lucio PS, Hannart A, Durand B, de Souza RN, Ribeiro ZM. The influence of local environment on the aging and mortality of *Aedes aegypti* (L.): case study in Fortaleza-CE, Brazil. *J Vector Ecol*. 2012;37(2):428–41, https://doi.org/10.1111/j.1948-7134.2012.00247.x

Donnelly MAP, Kluh S, Snyder RE, Barker CM. Quantifying sociodemographic heterogeneities in the distribution of *Aedes aegypti* among California households. *PLoS Negl Trop Dis*. 2020;14(7):e0008408, https://doi.org/10.1371/journal.pntd.0008408

Dunbar MW, Correa-Morales F, Dzul-Manzanilla F, Medina-Barreiro A, Bibiano-Marín W, Morales-Ríos E, et al. Efficacy of novel indoor residual spraying methods targeting pyrethroid-resistant *Aedes aegypti* within experimental houses. *PLoS Negl Trop Dis*. 2019;13(2):e0007203, https://doi.org/10.1371/journal.pntd.0007203

Duncombe J, Lau C, Weinstein P, Aaskov J, Rourke M, Grant R, et al. Seroprevalence of dengue in American Samoa, 2010. *Emerg Infect Dis*. 2013;19(2):324–6, https://doi.org/10.3201/eid1902.120464

Dzul-Manzanilla F, Correa-Morales F, Che-Mendoza A, Palacio-Vargas J, Sánchez-Tejeda G, González-Roldan JF, et al. Identifying urban hotspots of dengue, chikungunya, and Zika transmission in Mexico to support risk stratification efforts: a spatial analysis. *Lancet Planet Health*. 2021;5(5):e277–e85, https://doi.org/10.1016/S2542-5196(21)00030-9

Eamchan P, Nisalak A, Foy HM, Chareonsook OA. Epidemiology and control of dengue virus infections in Thai villages in 1987. *Am J Trop Med Hyg*. 1989;41:95–101, https://doi.org/10.4269/ajtmh.1989.41.95

Effler PV, Pang L, Kitsutani P, Vorndam V, Nakata M, Ayers T, Elm J, Tom T, Reiter P, Rigau-Perez JG, Hayes JM. Dengue fever, Hawaii, 2001-2002. *Emerg Infect Dis*. 2005;11(5):742–9, https://doi.org/10.3201/eid1105.041063

Ehrenkranz NJ, Ventura AK, Cuadrado RR, Pond WL, Porter JE. Pandemic dengue in Caribbean countries and the southern United States--past, present and potential problems. *N Engl J Med*. 1971;285(26):1460–9, https://doi.org/10.1056/NEJM197112232852606

Eiras AE, Buhagiar TS, Ritchie SA. Development of the gravid *Aedes* trap for the capture of adult female container-exploiting mosquitoes (Diptera: Culicidae). *J Med Entomol*. 2014;51(1):200–9, https://doi.org/10.1603/me13104

Endy TP, Anderson KB, Nisalak A, Yoon IK, Green S, Rothman AL, et al. Determinants of inapparent and symptomatic dengue infection in a prospective study of primary school children in Kamphaeng Phet, Thailand. *PLoS Negl Trop Dis*. 2011;5(3): e975, https://doi.org/10.1371/journal.pntd.0000975

EPA. Methoprene: Environmental Protection Agency;2025a [cited May 19, 2025]. Available from: https://search.epa.gov/epasearch/?querytext=meth oprene&areaname=&areacontacts=&areasearchurl=&typeofsearch=epa&result_template=#/.

EPA. U.S. Insect repellents: Environmental Protection Agency;2025b [cited 19 May 2025]. Available from: https://www.epa.gov/insect-repellents

Facchinelli L, Badolo A, McCall PJ. Biology and behaviour of *Aedes aegypti* in the human environment: opportunities for vector control of arbovirus transmission. *Viruses*. 2023;15(3):636, https://doi.org/10.3390/v15030636

Facchinelli L, Valerio L, Pombi M, Reiter P, Constantini C, Della Torre A. Development of a novel sticky trap for container breeding mosquitoes and evaluation of its sampling properties to monitor urban populations of *Aedes albopictus*. *Med Vet Entomol*. 2007;21:183–95, https://doi.org/10.1111/j.1365-2915.2007.00680.x

Farajollahi A, Price DC. A rapid identification guide for larvae of the most common North American container-inhabiting *Aedes* species of medical importance. *J Am Mosq Control Assoc*. 2013;29(3):203–21, https://doi.org/10.2987/11-6198R.1

Farajollahi A, Healy S, Unlu I, Gaugler R, Fonseca D. Effectiveness of ultra-low volume nighttime applications of an adulticide against diurnal *Aedes albopictus*, a critical vector of dengue and chikungunya viruses. *PLoS One*. 2012;7(11):e49181, https://doi.org/10.1371/journal.pone.0049181

Farajollahi A, Williams G, Condon G, Kesavaraju B, Unlu I, Gaugler R. Assessment of a direct application of two *Bacillus thuringiensis israelensis* formulations for immediate and residual control of *Aedes albopictus*. *J Am Mosq Control Assoc*. 2013;29(4):385–8, https://doi.org/10.2987/13-6332.1

Farajollahi A, Kesavaraju B, Price DC, Williams GM, Healy SP, Gaugler R, et al. Field efficacy of BG-Sentinel and industry-standard traps for *Aedes albopictus* (Diptera: Culicidae) and West Nile virus surveillance. *J Med Entomol*. 2009;46(4):919–25, https://doi.org/10.1603/033.046.0426

Fay RW. A trap based on visual responses of adult mosquitoes. *Mosq News*. 1968;28:1–7.

Fay RW, Eliason DA. A preferred oviposition site as a surveillance method for *Aedes aegypti*. *Mosq News*. 1966;26(4):531–5.

Fay RW, Prince WH. A modified visual trap for *Aedes aegypti*. *Mosq News*. 1970;30(1):20–3.

Fitzmaurice GM, Laird NM, Ware JW. *Applied Longitudinal Analysis* (Boston, MA: John Wiley & Sons, 2011, p. 701).

Flores A, Ponce G, Silva B, Gutierrez S, Bobadilla C, Lopez B, et al. Widespread cross resistance to pyrethroids in *Aedes aegypti* (Diptera: Culicidae) from Veracruz state Mexico. *J Econom Entomol*. 2013;106(2):959–69, https://doi.org/10.1603/ec12284

FMEL. Florida Medical Entomology Laboratory. Mosquito guide [Internet]. University of Florida; [cited 19 May 2025], https://fmel.ifas.ufl.edu/mosquito-guide/

Focks DA. *A Review of Entomological Sampling Methods and Indicators for Dengue Vectors* (Geneva, Switzerland: TDR/WHO, TDR/IDE/DEN/03.1. 2003), https://iris.who.int/bitstream/handle/10665/204934/B0219.pdf?sequence=1#page=233

Focks D. *Toxorhynchites* as biocontrol agents. *J Am Mosq Control Assoc*. 2007;23(suppl 2):118–27, https://doi.org/10.2987/8756-971x(2007)23[118:taba]2.0.co;2

Focks DA, Bangs MJ, Churchc C, Juffried M, Sustriayu Nalime S. Transmission thresholds and pupal/demographic surveys in Yogyakarta, Indonesia for developing a dengue control strategy based on targeting epidemiologically significant types of water-holding containers. *Dengue Bull*. 2007;31:83–102.

Focks D, Barrera R. *Dengue Transmission Dynamics: Assessment and Implications for Control* (Geneva, Switzerland: TDR/WHO, 2007).

Focks DA, Brenner RJ, Hayes J, Daniels E. Transmission thresholds for dengue in terms of *Aedes aegypti* pupae per person with discussion of their utility in source reduction efforts. *Am J Trop Med Hyg*. 2000;62(1):11–8, https://doi.org/10.4269/ajtmh.2000.62.11

Focks DA, Chadee DD. Pupal survey: An epidemiologically significant surveillance method for *Aedes aegypti*: An example using data from Trinidad. *Am J Trop Med Hyg*. 1997;56(2):159–67, https://doi.org/10.4269/ajtmh.1997.56.159

Fonseca DM, Unlu I, Crepeau T, Farajollahi A, Healy SP, Bartlett-Healy K, et al. Area-wide management of *Aedes albopictus*. Part 2: Gauging the efficacy of traditional integrated pest control measures against urban container mosquitoes. *Pest Manag Sci*. 2013. 69(12):1351–61, https://doi.org/10.1002/ps.3511

Fontoura N, Bellinato D, Valle D, Pereira Lima J. The efficacy of a chitin synthesis inhibitor against field populations of organophosphate-resistant *Aedes aegypti* in Brazil. *Mem Inst Oswaldo Cruz*. 2012;107(3):387–95, https://doi.org/10.1590/s0074-02762012000300014

Franz AW, Clem RJ, Passarelli AL. Novel genetic and molecular tools for the investigation and control of dengue virus transmission by mosquitoes. *Curr Trop Med Rep*. 2014;1(1):21–31, https://doi.org/10.1007/s40475-013-0007-2

Freier JE, Francy DB. A duplex cone trap for the collection of adult *Aedes albopictus*. *J Am Mosq Control Assoc*. 1991;7(1):73–9.

Garcia-Rejon J, Lorono-Pino MA, Farfan-Ale JA, Flores-Flores L, Rosado-Paredes ED, Rivero-Cardenas N, et al. Dengue virus-infected *Aedes aegypti* in the home environment. *Am J Trop Med Hyg*. 2008;79(6):940–50, https://doi.org/10.4269/ajtmh.2008.79.940

Garcia-Rejon JE, Lorono-Pino MA, Farfan-Ale JA, Flores-Flores LF, Lopez-Uribe MP, Najera-Vazquez MD, et al. Mosquito infestation and dengue virus infection in *Aedes aegypti* females in schools in Merida, Mexico. *Am J Trop Med Hyg*. 2011;84(3):489–96, https://doi.org/10.4269/ajtmh.2011.10-0654

Garcia KKS, Versiani HS, Araújo TO, Conceição JPA, Obara MT, Ramalho WM, et al. Measuring mosquito control: adult-mosquito catches vs egg-trap data as endpoints of a cluster-randomized controlled trial of mosquito-disseminated pyriproxyfen. *Parasit Vectors*. 2020;13(1):352, https://doi.org/10.1186/s13071-020-04221-z

Garza-Robledo AA, Martinez-Perales JF, Rodriguez-Castro VA, Quiroz-Martinez H. Effectiveness of spinosad and temephos for the control of mosquito larvae at a tire dump in Allende, Nuevo Leon, Mexico. *J Am Mosq Control Assoc*. 2011;27(4):404–7, https://doi.org/10.2987/11-6133.1

Getis A, Morrison AC, Gray K, Scott TW. Characteristics of the spatial pattern of the dengue vector, *Aedes aegypti*, in Iquitos, Peru. *Am J Trop Med Hyg*. 2003;69(5):494–505, https://doi.org/10.4269/ajtmh.2003.69.494

Gilbertson WE. Sanitary aspects of the control of the 1943-1944 epidemic of dengue fever in Honolulu. [not specified]. *Am J Public Health*. 1945;35(3):261-270, https://doi.org/http://dx.doi.org/10.2105/AJPH.35.3.261

Gill SS, Cowles EA, Pietrantonio PV. The mode of action of *Bacillus thuringiensis* endotoxins. *Ann Rev Entomol.* 1992;37:615–36, https://doi.org/10.1146/annurev.en.37.010192.003151

Gloria-Soria A, Faraji A, Hamik J, White G, Amsberry S, Donahue M, et al. Origins of high latitude introductions of *Aedes aegypti* to Nebraska and Utah during 2019. *Infect Genet Evol.* 2022;103:105333, https://doi.org/10.1016/j.meegid.2022.105333

Gomes ADC, Da Silva NN, Bernal RTI, Leandro ADS, De Camargo NJ, Da Silva AM, et al. Specificity of the Adultrap for capturing females of *Aedes aegypti* (Diptera: Culicidae). [Portuguese]. *Rev Soc Brasileira Med Trop.* 2007;40(2):216–9, https://doi.org/10.1590/s0037-86822007000200014

Gonzalez Obando R, Gamboa F, Perafan O, Suarez MF, Montoya J. Experiencia de un análisis entomológico de criaderos de *Aedes aegypti* y *Culex quinquefasciatus* en Cali, Colombia. *Rev Colomb Entomol.* 2007;33:148–56, http://www.scielo.org.co/scielo.php?script=sci_arttext&pid=S0120-04882007000200011&lng=en&nrm=iso>. ISSN 0120-0488

Gratz NG. Critical review of the vector status of *Aedes albopictus. Med Vet Entomol.* 2004;18(3):215–27, https://doi.org/10.1111/j.0269-283X.2004.00513.x

Grieco JP, Achee NL, Chareonviriyaphap T, Suwonkerd W, Chauhan K, Sardelis MR, et al. A new classification system for the actions of IRS chemicals traditionally used for malaria control. *PLoS One.* 2007;2(8):e716, https://doi.org/10.1371/journal.pone.0000716

Gubler DJ. Dengue. In: Monath TP, editor. *The Arboviruses: Epidemiology and Ecology* (Boca Raton, FL: CRC Press, 1988).

Gubler DJ, Novak RJ, Vergne E, Colon NA, Velez M, Fowler J. *Aedes* (*Gymnometopa*) *mediovittatus* (Diptera: Culicidae), a potential maintenance vector of dengue viruses in Puerto Rico. *J Med Entomol.* 1985;22(5):469–75, https://doi.org/10.1093/jmedent/22.5.469

Hahn MB, Eisen L, McAllister J, Savage HM, Mutebi JP, Eisen RJ. Updated reported distribution of *Aedes* (*Stegomyia*) *aegypti* and *Aedes* (*Stegomyia*) *albopictus* (Diptera: Culicidae) in the United States, 1995-2016. *J Med Entomol.* 2017;54(5):1420–4, https://doi.org/10.1093/jme/tjx088

Halstead SB, Scanlon JE, Umpaivit P, Udomsakdi S. Dengue and chikungunya virus infection in man in Thailand, 1962-1964. IV. Epidemiologic studies in the Bangkok metropolitan area. *Am J Trop Med Hyg.* 1969;18(6):997–1021, https://doi.org/10.4269/ajtmh.1969.18.997

Hapairai LK, Mysore K, James LD, Scheel ND, Realey JS, Sun L, et al. Evaluation of large volume yeast interfering RNA lure-and-kill ovitraps for attraction and control of *Aedes* mosquitoes. *Med Vet Entomol.* 2021;35(3):361–70, https://doi.org/10.1111/mve.12504

Harrison BA, Callahan MC, Watts DM, Panthusiri L. An efficient floating larval trap for sampling *Aedes aegypti* populations (Diptera: Culicidae). *J Med Entomol*. 1982;19:722–7, https://doi.org/10.1093/jmedent/19.6.722

Hasty JM, Felix GE, Amador M, Barrera R, Santiago GS, Nakasone L, Park SY, Okoji S, Honda E, Asuncion B, Save M. Entomological investigation detects dengue virus Type 1 in *Aedes* (*Stegomyia*) *albopictus* (Skuse) during the 2015-16 outbreak in Hawaii. *Am J Trop Med Hyg*. 2020;102(4):869–75, https://doi.org/10.4269/ajtmh.19-0732

Hawley WA. The biology of *Aedes albopictus*. *J Am Mosq Control Assoc*. 1988;4(1):1–40.

Hayes JM, Rigau-Pérez JG, Reiter P, Effler PV, Pang L, Vorndam V, Hinten SR, Mark KE, Myers MF, Street K, Bergau L. Risk factors for infection during a dengue-1 outbreak in Maui, Hawaii, 2001. *Trans R Soc Trop Med Hyg*. 2006;100(6):559–66, https://doi.org/10.1016/j.trstmh.2005.08.013

Hayes RO, Kitaguchi GE, Mann RM. The CDC sweeper a six volt mechanical aspirator for collecting adult mosquitoes. *Mosq News*. 1967;27:359–63.

Healy JM, Burgess MC, Chen TH, Hancock WT, Toews KE, Anesi MS, et al. Notes from the field: Outbreak of Zika virus disease - American Samoa, 2016. *MMWR Morb Mortal Wkly Rep*. 2016;65(41):1146–7, https://doi.org/10.15585/mmwr.mm6541a4

Hemme RR, Smith EA, Felix G, White BJ, Diaz-Garcia MI, Rodriguez D, et al. Multi-year mass-trapping with autocidal gravid ovitraps has limited influence on insecticide susceptibility in *Aedes aegypti* (Diptera: Culicidae) from Puerto Rico. *J Med Entomol*. 2022;59(1):314–9, https://doi.org/10.1093/jme/tjab162

Hemme RR, Vizcaino L, Harris AF, Felix G, Kavanaugh M, Kenney JL, et al. Rapid screening of *Aedes aegypti* mosquitoes for susceptibility to insecticides as part of Zika emergency response, Puerto Rico. *Emerg Infect Dis*. 2019;25(10):1959–61, https://doi.org/10.3201/eid2510.181847

Hernandez-Avila J, Rodriguez M-H, Sanchez Castaneda V, Roman Perez S, Rodriguez M-H, Santos Luna R, et al. Nation-wide, web-based, geographic information system for the integrated surveillance and control of dengue fever in Mexico. *PLoS One*. 2013;8(8):e70231, https://doi.org/10.1371/journal.pone.0070231

Hills SL, Piispanen JP, Humphreys JL, Foley PN. A focal, rapidly-controlled outbreak of dengue fever in two suburbs in Townsville, North Queensland, 2001. *Commun Dis Intell Q Rep*. 2002;26(4):596–600.

Hobbs JH, Hughes EA, Eichold BH, 2nd. Replacement of *Aedes aegypti* by *Aedes albopictus* in Mobile, Alabama. *J Am Mosq Control Assoc*. 1991;7(3):488–9.

Hoffmann AA, Montgomery BL, Popovici J, Iturbe-Ormaetxe I, Johnson PH, Muzzi F, et al. Successful establishment of *Wolbachia* in *Aedes* populations to suppress dengue transmission. *Nature*. 2011;476(7361):454–7, https://doi.org/10.1038/nature10356

Hopp MJ, Foley JA. Global-scale relationships between climate and the dengue fever vector, *Aedes aegypti*. *Clim Chang*. 2001;48:441–63.

Hribar LJ, Boehmler MB, Murray HL, Pruszynski CA, Leal AL. Mosquito surveillance and insecticide resistance monitoring conducted by the Florida Keys Mosquito Control District, Monroe County, Florida, USA. *Insects*. 2022;13(10):927, https://doi.org/10.3390/insects13100927

Hribar L, Whiteside M. Seasonal habitat use by immature *Aedes aegypti* (Linnaeus) (Diptera: Culicidae) in the Florida Keys, USA. *Stud Dipterologica*. 2010;17:237–51.

Huerta H, González-Roldán JF, Sánchez-Tejeda G, Correa-Morales F, Romero-Contreras FE, Cárdenas-Flores R, et al. Detection of Zika virus in *Aedes* mosquitoes from Mexico. *Trans R Soc Trop Med Hyg*. 2017;111(7):328–31, https://doi.org/10.1093/trstmh/trx056

Hugo LE, Cook PE, Johnson PH, Rapley LP, Kay BH, Ryan PA, Ritchie SA, O'Neill SL. Field validation of a transcriptional assay for the prediction of age of uncaged *Aedes aegypti* mosquitoes in Northern Australia. *PLoS Negl Trop Dis*. 2010;4(2):e608, https://doi.org/10.1371/journal.pntd.0000608

Hustedt JC, Boyce R, Bradley J, Hii J, Alexander N. Use of pyriproxyfen in control of *Aedes* mosquitoes: a systematic review. *PLoS Negl Trop Dis*. 2020;14(6):e0008205, https://doi.org/10.1371/journal.pntd.0008205

Indriani C, Tanamas SK, Khasanah U, Ansari MR, Rubangi, Tantowijoyo W, et al. Impact of randomised wmel *Wolbachia* deployments on notified dengue cases and insecticide fogging for dengue control in Yogyakarta City. *Glob Health Action*. 2023;16(1):2166650, https://doi.org/10.1080/16549716.2023.2166650

Iyaloo DP, Facknath S, Bheecarry A. Field evaluation of BG SentinelTM traps of four different black-and-white color combinations in Mauritius for enhanced *Ae. albopictus* mosquito collection. *Int J Mosq Res*. 2017;4:43–9.

Jachowski Jr LA. Filariasis in American Samoa. V. Bionomics of the principal vector, *Aedes polynesiensis* Marks. *Am J Epidemiol*. 1954;60(2):186–203, https://doi.org/10.1093/oxfordjournals.aje.a119712

Jacups SP, Ball TS, Paton CJ, Johnson PH, Ritchie SA. Operational use of household bleach to "crash and release" *Aedes aegypti* prior to *Wolbachia*-infected mosquito release. *J Med Entomol*. 2013a;50(2):344–51, https://doi.org/10.1603/me12043. PMID: 23540123

Jacups SP, Rapley LP, Johnson PH, Benjamin S, Ritchie SA. *Bacillus thuringiensis* var. *israelensis* misting for control of *Aedes* in cryptic ground containers in North Queensland, Australia. *Am J Trop Med Hyg*. 2013b;88(3):490–6, https://doi.org/10.4269/ajtmh.12-0385

Johansson MA, Dominici F, Glass GE. Local and global effects of climate on dengue transmission in Puerto Rico. *PLoS Negl Trop Dis*. 2009;3(2):e382, https://doi.org/10.1371/journal.pntd.0000382

Johnson BJ, Brosch D, Christiansen A, Wells E, Wells M, Bhandoola AF, et al. Neighbors help neighbors control urban mosquitoes. *Sci Rep*. 2018;8(1):15797, https://doi.org/10.1038/s41598-018-34161-9

Jones RC, Weaver KN, Smith S, Blanco C, Flores C, Gibbs K, et al. Use of the vector index and geographic information system to prospectively inform West Nile virus interventions. *J Am Mosq Control Assoc*. 2011;27(3):315–9, https://doi.org/10.2987/10-6098.1

Juarez JG, Chaves LF, Garcia-Luna SM, Martin E, Badillo-Vargas I, Medeiros MCI, et al. Variable coverage in an Autocidal Gravid Ovitrap intervention impacts efficacy of *Aedes aegypti* control. *J Appl Ecol*. 2021;58(10):2075–86, https://doi.org/10.1111/1365-2664.13951

Juliano SA. Species introduction and replacement among mosquitoes: interspecific resource competition or apparent competition? *Ecology*. 1998;79(1):255–68, https://doi.org/10.1890/0012-9658(1998)079[0255:SIARAM]2.0.CO;2

Jupp PG, Mclntosh BM. Chikungunya virus disease. In: Monath TP, editor. *The Arboviruses: Epidemiology and Ecology*, (Boca Raton, FL.: CRC Press, 1988), pp. 137–57.

Jury MR. Climate influence on dengue epidemics in Puerto Rico. *Int J Environ Health Res*. 2008;18(5):323–34, https://doi.org/10.1080/09603120701849836

Kan CC, Lee PF, Wen TH, Chao DY, Wu MH, Lin NH, et al. Two clustering diffusion patterns identified from the 2001-2003 dengue epidemic, Kaohsiung, Taiwan. *Am J Trop Med Hyg*. 2008;79(3):344–52, https://doi.org/10.4269/ajtmh.2008.79.344

Kay BH, Cabral CP, Araujo DB, Ribeiro ZM, Braga PH, Sleigh AC. Evaluation of a funnel trap for collecting copepods and immature mosquitos from wells. *J Am Mosq Control Assoc*. 1992;8(4):372–5.

Kay B, Nam VS. New strategy against *Aedes aegypti* in Vietnam. *Lancet*. 2005;365(9459):613–7, https://doi.org/10.1016/S0140-6736(05)17913-6

Kay BH, Ryan PA, Russell BM, Holt JS, Lyons SA, Foley PN. The importance of subterranean mosquito habitat to arbovirus vector control strategies in North Queensland, Australia. *J Med Entomol*. 2000;37:846–53, https://doi.org/10.1603/0022-2585-37.6.846

Kenney JL, Burkhalter KL, Scott ML, McAllister J, Lang FE, Webster S, et al. Entomological investigations during early stages of a chikungunya outbreak in the United States Virgin Islands, 2014. *J Am Mosq Control Assoc*. 2017;33(1):8–15, https://doi.org/10.2987/16-6619.1

Khan SU, Ogden NH, Fazil AA, Gachon PH, Dueymes GU, Greer AL, Ng V. Current and projected distributions of *Aedes aegypti* and *Ae. albopictus* in Canada and the U.S. *Environ Health Perspect.* 2020;128(5):57007, https://doi.org/10.1289/EHP5899

Kilpatrick AM, Pape WJ. Predicting human West Nile virus infections with mosquito surveillance data. *Am J Epidemiol.* 2013;178(5):829–35, https://doi.org/10.1093/aje/kwt046

Knols BG, Bukhari T, Farenhorst M. Entomopathogenic fungi as the next-generation control agents against malaria mosquitoes. *Future Microbiol.* 2010;5(3):339–41, https://doi.org/10.2217/fmb.10.11

Koyoc-Cardeña E, Medina-Barreiro A, Cohuo-Rodríguez A, Pavía-Ruz N, Lenhart A, Ayora-Talavera G, et al. Estimating absolute indoor density of *Aedes aegypti* using removal sampling. *Parasit Vectors.* 2019;12(1):250, https://doi.org/10.1186/s13071-019-3503-y

Kraemer MU, Reiner Jr RC, Brady OJ, Messina JP, Gilbert M, Pigott DM, Yi D, Johnson K, Earl L, Marczak LB, Shirude S. Past and future spread of the arbovirus vectors *Aedes aegypti* and *Aedes albopictus. Nat Microbiol.* 2019, https://doi.org/10.1038/s41564-019-0440-7

Kretschmer M, Collins J, Dale AP, Garrett B, Koski L, Zabel K, et al. Notes from the field: first evidence of locally acquired dengue virus infection - Maricopa County, Arizona, November 2022. *MMWR Morb Mortal Wkly Rep.* 2023;72(11):290–1, https://doi.org/10.15585/mmwr.mm7211a5

Krockel U, Rose A, Eiras AE, Geier M. New tools for surveillance of adult yellow fever mosquitoes: comparison of trap catches with human landing rates in an urban environment. *J Am Mosq Control Assoc.* 2006;22(2):229–38, https://doi.org/10.2987/8756-971X(2006)22[229:NTFSOA]2.0.CO;2

Kroeger A, Lenhart A, Ochoa M, Villegas E, Levy M, Alexander N, et al. Effective control of dengue vectors with curtains and water container covers treated with insecticide in Mexico and Venezuela: cluster randomised trials. *BMJ.* 2006;27;332(7552):1247–52, https://doi.org/10.1136/bmj.332.7552.1247

Lambrechts L, Scott TW, Gubler DJ. Consequences of the expanding global distribution of *Aedes albopictus* for dengue virus transmission. *PLoS Negl Trop Dis.* 2010;4(5):e646, https://doi.org/10.1371/journal.pntd.0000646

Leandro AS, Lopes RD, Amaral Martins C, Delai RM, Villela DAM, Maciel-de-Freitas R. Entomo-virological surveillance followed by serological active survey of symptomatic individuals is helpful to identify hotspots of early arbovirus transmission. *Front Public Health.* 2022;10:1024187, https://doi.org/10.3389/fpubh.2022.1024187

Lega J, Brown HE, Barrera R. A 70% reduction in mosquito populations does not require removal of 70% of mosquitoes. *J Med Entomol.* 2020;57(5):1668–70, https://doi.org/10.1093/jme/tjaa066

Linthicum KJ, Kramer VL, Madon MB, Fujioka K. Introduction and potential establishment of *Aedes albopictus* in California in 2001. *J Am Mosq Control Assoc.* 2003;19(4):301–8.

Little E, Barrera R, Seto K, Diuk-Wasser M. Co-occurrence patterns of the dengue vector *Aedes aegypti* and *Ae. mediovitattus*, a potential native dengue vector in Puerto Rico. *Am J Trop Med Hyg.* 2011;1):372, https://doi.org/10.1007/s10393-011-0708-8

Lloyd LS. *Best practices for dengue prevention and control in the Americas*, (Washington, DC: Environmental Health Project, USAID, 2003. Report No. 7).

Lorono-Pino MA, Garcia-Rejon JE, Machain-Williams C, Gomez-Carro S, Nunez-Ayala G, Najera-Vazquez Mdel R, et al. Towards a casa segura: a consumer product study of the effect of insecticide-treated curtains on *Aedes aegypti* and dengue virus infections in the home. *Am J Trop Med Hyg.* 2013;89(2):385–97, https://doi.org/10.4269/ajtmh.12-0772

Lounibos LP, Bargielowski I, Carrasquilla MC, Nishimura N. Coexistence of *Aedes aegypti* and *Aedes albopictus* (Diptera: Culicidae) in Peninsular Florida two decades after competitive displacements. *J Med Entomol.* 2016;53(6):1385–90, https://doi.org/10.1093/jme/tjw122

Lozano-Fuentes S, Hayden MH, Welsh-Rodriguez C, Ochoa-Martinez C, Tapia-Santos B, Kobylinski KC, Uejio CK, Zielinski-Gutierrez E, Delle Monache L, Monaghan AJ, Steinhoff DF. The dengue virus mosquito vector *Aedes aegypti* at high elevation in Mexico. *Am J Trop Med Hyg.* 2012;87(5):902–9, https://doi.org/10.4269/ajtmh.2012.12-0244

Luce R, Rivera A, Mohammed H, Tomashek KM, Lehman J. Travel-associated dengue surveillance - United States, 2006-2008. *MMWR Morb Mortal Wkly Rep.* 2010;18;59(23):715–9.

Lumsdex WHR. An epidemic of virus disease in Southern Province, Tanganyika Territory in 1952-53. *Trans R Soc Trop Med Hyg.* 1955;49:33–57, https://doi.org/10.1016/0035-9203(55)90080-8.

Maciel-De-Freitas R, Codeco CT, Lourenco-De-Oliveira R. Daily survival rates and dispersal of *Aedes aegypti* females in Rio de Janeiro, Brazil. *Am J Trop Med Hyg.* 2007;76(4):659–65, https://doi.org/10.4269/ajtmh.2007.76.659

Maciel-de-Freitas R, Eiras AE, Lourenco-de-Oliveira R. Field evaluation of effectiveness of the BG-Sentinel, a new trap for capturing adult *Aedes aegypti* (Diptera: Culicidae). *Mem Inst Oswaldo Cruz.* 2006;101(3):321–5, https://doi.org/10.1590/s0074-02762006000300017

Mackay A, Amador M, Barrera R. An improved autocidal gravid ovitrap for the control and surveillance of *Aedes aegypti*. *Parasit Vectors.* 2013;6(1):225, https://doi.org/10.1186/1756-3305-6-225

Mackay AJ, Amador M, Felix G, Acevedo V, Barrera R. Evaluation of household bleach as an ovicide for the control of *Aedes aegypti. J Am Mosq Control Assoc.* 2015;31(1):77–84, https://doi.org/10.2987/14-6427R.1

Madewell ZJ, Hemme RR, Adams L, Barrera R, Waterman SH, Johansson MA. Comparing vector and human surveillance strategies to detect arbovirus transmission: a simulation study for Zika virus detection in Puerto Rico. *PLoS Negl Trop Dis.* 2019;13(12):e0007988, https://doi.org/10.1371/journal.pntd.0007988

Madon MB, Hazelrigg JE, Shaw MW, Kluh S, Mulla. Has *Aedes albopictus* established in California? *J Am Mosq Control Assoc.* 2003;19(4):297–300

Mains JW, Kelly PH, Dobson KL, Petrie WD, Dobson SL. Localized control of *Aedes aegypti* (Diptera: Culicidae) in Miami, FL, via inundative releases of *Wolbachia*-Infected male mosquitoes. *J Med Entomol.* 2019;56(5):1296–303, https://doi.org/10.1093/jme/tjz051

Mani TR, Arunachalam N, Rajendran R, Satyanarayana K, Dash AP. Efficacy of thermal fog application of deltacide, a synergized mixture of pyrethroids, against *Aedes aegypti*, the vector of dengue. *Trop Med Int Health.* 2005;10(12):1298–304, https://doi.org/10.1111/j.1365-3156.2005.01522.x

Manrique-Saide P, Arisqueta-Chablé C, Geded-Moreno E, Herrera-Bójorquez J, Uc V, Chablé-Santos J, et al. An assessment of the importance of subsurface catch basins for *Aedes aegypti* adult production during the dry season in a neighborhood of Merida, Mexico. *J Am Mosq Control Assoc.* 2013;29:164–7, https://doi.org/10.2987/12-6320R.1

Manrique-Saide P, Herrera-Bójorquez J, Medina-Barreiro A, Trujillo-Peña E, Villegas-Chim J, Valadez-González N, et al. Insecticide-treated house screening protects against Zika-infected *Aedes aegypti* in Merida, Mexico. *PLoS Negl Trop Dis.* 2021;15(1):e0009005, https://doi.org/10.1371/journal.pntd.0009005

Marcombe S, Farajollahi A, Healy SP, Clark GG, Fonseca DM. Insecticide resistance status of United States populations of *Aedes albopictus* and mechanisms involved. *PLoS One.* 2014;9(7):e101992, https://doi.org/10.1371/journal.pone.0101992

Marten GG. Elimination of *Aedes albopictus* from tire piles by introducing *Macrocyclops albidus* (Copepoda, Cyclopidae). *J Am Mosq Control Assoc.* 1990;6(4):689–93.

Marten GG, Caballero X, Larios A, Bendaña H. Proof of concept for eliminating *Aedes aegypti* production by means of integrated control including turtles, copepods, tilapia, larvicides, and community participation in Monte Verde, Honduras. *Acta Trop.* 2022;227:106269, https://doi.org/10.1016/j.actatropica.2021.106269

Marten GG, Reid JW. Cyclopoid copepods. *J Am Mosq Control Assoc.* 2007;23(2):65–92.

Mavale M, Sudeep A, Gokhale M, Hundekar S, Parashar D, Ghodke Y, et al. Persistence of viral RNA in chikungunya virus-infected *Aedes aegypti* (Diptera: Culicidae) mosquitoes after prolonged storage at 28°C. *Am J Trop Med Hyg.* 2012;86(1):178–80, https://doi.org/10.4269/ajtmh.2012.11-0236

McGregor BL, Connelly CR. A Review of the control of *Aedes aegypti* (Diptera: Culicidae) in the continental United States. *J Med Entomol.* 2021;58(1):10–25, https://doi.org/10.1093/jme/tjaa157

McHugh CP. Distributional records from the U.S. Air Force ovitrapping programme - 1990. *J Am Mosq Control Assoc.* 1991;7(3):499–501.

Meeraus WH, Armistead JS, Arias JR. Field comparison of novel and gold standard traps for collecting *Aedes albopictus* in Northern Virginia. *J Am Mosq Control Assoc.* 2008;24(2):244–8, https://doi.org/10.2987/5676.1

Mendez F, Barreto M, Arias JF, Rengifo G, Munoz J, Burbano ME, et al. Human and mosquito infections by dengue viruses during and after epidemics in a dengue-endemic region of Colombia. *Am J Trop Med Hyg.* 2006;74(4):678–83, https://doi.org/10.4269/ajtmh.2006.74.678

Mercer DR, Marie J, Bossin H, Faaruia M, Tetuanui A, Sang MC, et al. Estimation of population size and dispersal of *Aedes polynesiensis* on Toamaro Motu, French Polynesia. *J Med Entomol.* 2012;49(5):971–80, https://doi.org/10.1603/me11234

Metzger ME, Hardstone Yoshimizu M, Padgett KA, Hu R, Kramer VL. Detection and establishment of *Aedes aegypti* and *Aedes albopictus* (Diptera: Culicidae) mosquitoes in California, 2011-2015. *J Med Entomol.* 2017;54(3):533–43, https://doi.org/10.1093/jme/tjw237

Mitchell CJ, Savage HM, Smith GC, Flood SP, Castro LT, Roppul M. Japanese encephalitis on Saipan: a survey of suspected mosquito vectors. *Am J Trop Med Hyg.* 1993;48(4):585–90, https://doi.org/10.4269/ajtmh.1993.48.585

Mogi M, Armbruster P, Fonseca DM. Analyses of the northern distributional limit of *Aedes albopictus* (Diptera: Culicidae) with a simple thermal index. *J Med Entomol.* 2012;49(6):1233–43, https://doi.org/10.1603/me12104

Mogi M, Choochote W, Khamboonruang C, Suwanpanit P. Applicability of presence-absence and sequential sampling for ovitrap surveillance of *Aedes* (Diptera: Culicidae) in Chiang Mai, Northern Thailand. *J Med Entomol.* 1990;27:509–14, https://doi.org/10.1093/jmedent/27.4.509

Monaghan AJ, Eisen RJ, Eisen L, McAllister J, Savage HM, Mutebi JP, et al. Consensus and uncertainty in the geographic range of *Aedes aegypti* and *Aedes albopictus* in the contiguous United States: multi-model assessment and synthesis. *PLoS Comput Biol.* 2019;15(10):e1007369, https://doi.org/10.1371/journal.pcbi.1007369, https://doi.org/10.1371/journal.pcbi.1007369

Monaghan AJ, Morin CW, Steinhoff DF, Wilhelmi O, Hayden M, Quattrochi DA, Reiskind M, Lloyd AL, Smith K, Schmidt CA, Scalf PE. On the seasonal occurrence and abundance of the Zika virus vector mosquito *Aedes aegypti* in the contiguous United States. *PLoS Curr*. 2016;8:ecurrents.outbreaks.50df c7f46798675fc63e7d7da563da76, https://doi.org/10.1371/currents.outbreak s.50dfc7f46798675fc63e7d7da563da76

Montgomery BL, Ritchie SA. Roof gutters: A key container for *Aedes aegypti* and *Ochlerotatus notoscriptus* (Diptera : Culicidae) in Australia. *Am J Trop Med Hyg*. 2002;67(3):244–6, https://doi.org/10.4269/ajtmh.2002.67.244

Moore CG. *Aedes albopictus* in the United States: current status and prospects for further spread. *J Am Mosq Control Assoc*. 1999;15(2):221–7.

Moore CG, Cline BL, Ruiz-Tibén E, Lee D, Romney-Joseph H, Rivera-Correa E. *Aedes aegypti* in Puerto Rico: environmental determinants of larval abundance and relation to dengue virus transmission *Am J Trop Med Hyg*. 1978;27(6):1225–31, https://doi.org/10.4269/ajtmh.1978.27.1225

Morens DM, Rigau-Perez JG, Lopez-Correa RH. Dengue in Puerto Rico, 1977: public health response to characterize and control an epidemic of multiple serotypes. *Am J Trop Med Hyg*. 1986;35(1):197–211, https://doi.org/10.4269/ajtmh.1986.35.197

Morrison AC, Costero A, Edman JD, Clark GG, Scott TW. Increased fecundity of *Aedes aegypti* fed human blood before release in a mark-recapture study in Puerto Rico. *J Am Mosq Control Assoc*. 1999;15(2):98–104.

Morrison AC, Reiner Jr RC, Elson WH, Astete H, Guevara C, Del Aguila C, et al. Efficacy of a spatial repellent for control of *Aedes*-borne virus transmission: A cluster-randomized trial in Iquitos, Peru. *Proc Natl Acad Sci U S A*. 2022;119(26):e2118283119, https://doi.org/10.1073/pnas.2118283119

Mulla MS. The future of insect growth regulators in vector control. *J Am Mosq Control Assoc*. 1995;11(2 Pt 2):269–73.

Mulla M, Thavara U, Tawatsin A, Chompoosri J, Zaim M, Su T. Laboratory and field evaluation of novaluron, a new acylurea insect growth regulator, against *Aedes aegypti* (Diptera: Culicidae). *J Vector Ecol*. 2003;28(2):241–54.

Muller D, Frentiu F, Rojas A, Moreira L, O'Neill S, Young P. A portable approach for the surveillance of dengue virus-infected mosquitoes. *J Virol Methods*. 2012;183(1):90–3, https://doi.org/10.1016/j.jviromet.2012.03.033

Murray KO, Rodriguez LF, Herrington E, Kharat V, Vasilakis N, Walker C, et al. Identification of dengue fever cases in Houston, Texas, with evidence of autochthonous transmission between 2003 and 2005. *Vector Borne Zoonotic Dis*. 2013;13:1–11, https://doi.org/10.1089/vbz.2013.1413

Musso D, Gubler DJ. Zika virus. *Clin Microbiol Rev*. 2016;29(3):487–524, https://doi.org/10.1128/CMR.00072-15

Mutebi JP, Wilke AB, Ostrum E, Vasquez C, Cardenas G, Carvajal A, Moreno M, Petrie WD, Rodriguez A, Presas H, Rodriguez J. Diel activity patterns of two distinct populations of *Aedes aegypti* in Miami, FL and Brownsville, TX. *Sci Rep.* 2022;12(1):5315, https://doi.org/10.1038/s41598-022-06586-w

Mysore K, Hapairai LK, Sun L, Li P, Wang CW, Scheel ND, et al. Characterization of a dual-action adulticidal and larvicidal interfering RNA pesticide targeting the Shaker gene of multiple disease vector mosquitoes. *PLoS Negl Trop Dis.* 2020;14(7):e0008479, https://doi.org/10.1371/journal. pntd.0008479

Nam VS, Yen NT, Kay BH, Marten GG, Reid JW. Eradication of *Aedes aegypti* from a village in Vietnam, using copepods and community participation. *Am J Trop Med Hyg.* 1998;59(4):657–60, https://doi.org/10.4269/ ajtmh.1998.59.657

Namias A, Jobe NB, Paaijmans KP, Huijben S. The need for practical insecticide-resistance guidelines to effectively inform mosquito-borne disease control programmes. *Elife.* 2021;10:e65655, https://doi.org/10.7554/ eLife.65655

Naranjo D, Qualls W, Mueller G, Samson D, Roque D, Alimi T, et al. Evaluation of boric acid sugar baits against *Aedes albopictus* (Diptera: Culicidae) in tropical environments. *Parasit Res.* 2013;112(4):1583–7, https://doi. org/10.1007/s00436-013-3312-8

Nathan MB, Focks DA. Pupal/demographic surveys to inform dengue-vector control. *Ann Trop Med Parasitol.* 2006;100:S1–3, https://doi. org/10.1179/136485906X105462

Nawrocki SJ, Hawley WA. Estimation of the northern limits of distribution of *Aedes albopictus* in North America. *J Am Mosq Control Assoc.* 1987;3(2):314–7.

Nayar J, Ali A. A review of monomolecular surface films as larvicides and pupicides of mosquitoes. *J Vector Ecol.* 2003;28(2):190–9.

Nelder M, Kesavaraju B, Farajollahi A, Healy S, Unlu I, Crepeau T, et al. Suppressing *Aedes albopictus*, an emerging vector of dengue and chikungunya viruses, by a novel combination of a monomolecular film and an insect-growth regulator. *Am J Trop Med Hyg.* 2010;82(5):831–7, https:// doi.org/10.4269/ajtmh.2010.09-0546

Newton EA, Reiter P. A model of the transmission of dengue fever with an evaluation of the impact of ultra-low volume (ULV) insecticide applications on dengue epidemics. *Am J Trop Med Hyg.* 1992;47(6):709–20, https://doi. org/10.4269/ajtmh.1992.47.709

Niebylski ML, Savage HM, Nasci RS, Craig Jr GB. Blood hosts of *Aedes albopictus* in the United States. *J Am Mosq Control Assoc.* 1994;10(3):447–50.

O'Connor L, Plichart C, Sang AC, Brelsfoard CL, Bossin HC, Dobson SL. Open release of male mosquitoes infected with a *Wolbachia* biopesticide: field performance and infection containment. *PLoS Negl Trop Dis.* 2012;6(11):e1797, https://doi.org/10.1371/journal.pntd.0001797

Obenauer PJ, Allan SA, Kaufman PE. *Aedes albopictus* (Diptera: Culicidae) oviposition response to organic infusions from common flora of suburban Florida. *J Vector Ecol*. 2010;35(2):301–6, https://doi.org/10.1111/j.1948-7134.2010.00086.x

Omeara GF, Evans LF, Gettman AD, Cuda JP. Spread of *Aedes albopictus* and decline of *Aedes aegypti* (Diptera, Culicidae) in Florida. *J Med Entomol*. 1995;32(4):554–62, https://doi.org/10.1093/jmedent/32.4.554

Omeara GF, Gettman AD, Evans LF, Scheel FD. Invasion of cemeteries in Florida by *Aedes albopictus*. *J Am Mosq Control Assoc*. 1992;8(1):1–10.

Ong J, Chong CS, Yap G, Lee C, Abdul Razak MA, Chiang S, et al. Gravitrap deployment for adult *Aedes aegypti* surveillance and its impact on dengue cases. *PLoS Negl Trop Dis*. 2020;14(8):e0008528, https://doi.org/10.1371/journal.pntd.0008528

PAHO. *Handbook for Integrated Vector Management in the Americas* (Washington, DC: PAHO, 2019a). [cited May 19, 2025]. Available from: https://iris.paho.org/bitstream/handle/10665.2/51759/Manejo%20Integrado_ENG_FINAL3.pdf?sequence=1&isAllowed=y

PAHO. *Manual for Indoor Residual Spraying in Urban Areas for Aedes aegypti Control*, (Washington, DC: PAHO, 2019b). [cited May 19, 2025]. Available from: https://iris.paho.org/handle/10665.2/51637

PAHO. *Dengue and Dengue Hemorrhagic Fever in the Americas: Guidelines for Prevention and Control* (Washington, DC: PAHO, 1994, p. 98). [cited May 19, 2025]. Available from: https://iris.paho.org/handle/10665.2/40300

PAHO. Data - National Dengue fever cases 2025. [cited May 19, 2025]. Available from: https://www3.paho.org/data/index.php/en/mnu-topics/indicadores-dengue-en/dengue-nacional-en/252-dengue-pais-ano-en.html.

Parker C, Ramirez D, Thomas C, Connelly CR. Baseline susceptibility status of Florida populations of *Aedes aegypti* (Diptera: Culicidae) and *Aedes albopictus*. *J Med Entomol*. 2020;57(5):1550–9, https://doi.org/10.1093/jme/tjaa068

Peacock BE, Smith JP, Gregory PG, Loyless TM, Mulrennen JJ, Simmonds PR, Padgett LJ, Cook EK, Eddins TR. *Aedes albopictus* in Florida. *J Am Mosq Control Assoc*. 1988;4(3):362–5.

Pena CJ, Gonzalvez G, Chadee DD. A modified tire ovitrap for the surveillance of *Aedes albopictus* in the field. *J Vector Ecol*. 2004;29:374–5.

Perich MJ, Bunner BL, Tidwell MA, Williams DC, Mara CD, Carvalhe T, et al. Penetration of ultra-low volume applied insecticide into dwellings for dengue vector control. *J Am Mosq Control Assoc*. 1992;8(2):137–42.

Perich MJ, Kardec A, Braga IA, Portal IF, Burge R, Zeichner BC, et al. Field evaluation of a lethal ovitrap against dengue vectors in Brazil. *Med Vet Entomol.* 2003;17(2):205–10, https://doi.org/10.1046/j.1365-2915.2003.00427.x

Perich MJ, Tidwell MA, Dobson SE, Sardelis MR, Zaglul A, Williams DC. Barrier spraying to control the malaria vector *Anopheles albimanus*: laboratory and field evaluation in the Dominican Republic. *Med Vet Entomol.* 1993;7(4):363–8, https://doi.org/10.1111/j.1365-2915.1993.tb00706.x

Pilger D, De Maesschalck M, Horstick O, San Martin JL. Dengue outbreak response: documented effective interventions and evidence gaps. *TropIKA.net.* 2010;1(1), https://journal.tropika.net/scielo.php?script=sci_arttext&pid=S2078-86062010000100002&lng=en

Pilger D, Lenhart A, Manrique-Saide P, Siqueira JB, da Rocha WT, Kroeger A. Is routine dengue vector surveillance in central Brazil able to accurately monitor the *Aedes aegypti* population? Results from a pupal productivity survey. *Trop Med Int Health.* 2011;16(9):1143–50, https://doi.org/10.1111/j.1365-3156.2011.02818.x

Pless E, Gloria-Soria A, Evans BR, Kramer V, Bolling BG, Tabachnick WJ, et al. Multiple introductions of the dengue vector, *Aedes aegypti*, into California. *PLoS Negl Trop Dis.* 2017;11(8):e0005718, https://doi.org/10.1371/journal.pntd.0005718

Pontes RJS, Freeman J, Oliveira-Lima JW, Hodgson JC, Spielman A. Vector densities that potentiate dengue outbreaks in a Brazilian city. *Am J Trop Med Hyg.* 2000;62(3):378–83, https://doi.org/10.4269/ajtmh.2000.62.378

Porcasi X, Rotela CH, Introini MV, Frutos N, Lanfri S, Peralta G, et al. An operative dengue risk stratification system in Argentina based on geospatial technology. *Geospat Health.* 2012;6(3):S31–42, https://doi.org/10.4081/gh.2012.120

Pruszynski CA, Hribar LJ, Mickle R, Leal AL. A Large scale biorational approach using *Bacillus thuringiensis israeliensis* (Strain AM65-52) for nanaging *Aedes aegypti* populations to prevent dengue, chikungunya and Zika transmission. *PLoS One.* 2017;12(2):e0170079, https://doi.org/10.1371/journal.pone.0170079

Radke EG, Gregory CJ, Kintziger KW, Sauber-Schatz EK, Hunsperger EA, Gallagher GR, et al. Dengue outbreak in Key West, Florida, USA, 2009. *Emerg Infect Dis.* 2012;18(1):135–7, https://doi.org/10.3201/eid1801.110130

Ramlee S, Mohd S-A. Odonata nymphs as potential biocontrol agent of mosquito larvae in Malaysia. *Southeast Asian J Trop Med Public Health.* 2022;53(4):426–35.

Ramos MM, Mohammed H, Zielinski-Gutierrez E, Hayden MH, Lopez JL, Fournier M, Trujillo AR, Burton R, Brunkard JM, Anaya-Lopez L, Banicki AA. Epidemic dengue and dengue hemorrhagic fever at the Texas-Mexico border: results of a household-based seroepidemiologic survey, December

2005. *Am J Trop Med Hyg*. 2008;78(3):364–9, https://doi.org/10.4269/ajtmh.2008.78.364

Ranson H, Burhani J, Lumjuan N, Black IV WC. Insecticide resistance in dengue vectors. *TropIKA.net*. 2010;1, http://journal.tropika.net/scielo.php?script=sci_arttext&pid=S2078-86062010000100003&nrm=iso

Rapley LP, Johnson PH, Williams CR, Silcock RM, Larkman M, Long SA, et al. A lethal ovitrap-based mass trapping scheme for dengue control in Australia: II. Impact on populations of the mosquito *Aedes aegypti*. *Med Vet Entomol*. 2009;23(4):303–16, https://doi.org/10.1111/j.1365-2915.2009.00834.x

Regis L, Monteiro AM, de Melo-Santos MAV, Silveira JC, Furtado AF, Acioli RV, et al. Developing new approaches for detecting and preventing *Aedes aegypti* population outbreaks: basis for surveillance, alert and control system. *Mem Inst Oswaldo Cruz*. 2008;103(1):50–9, https://doi.org/10.1590/s0074-02762008000100008

Reiner Jr RC, Stoddard ST, Vazquez-Prokopec GM, Astete H, Perkins TA, Sihuincha M, et al. Estimating the impact of city-wide *Aedes aegypti* population control: an observational study in Iquitos, Peru. *PLoS Negl Trop Dis*. 2019;13(5):e0007255, https://doi.org/10.1371/journal.pntd.0007255

Reisen WK, Basio RG. Oviposition trap surveys conducted on four USAF installations in the Western Pacific. *Mosq News*. 1972;32(1):107–8.

Reiter P, Amador MA, Colon N. Enhancement of the CDC ovitrap with hay infusions for daily monitoring of *Aedes aegypti* populations. *J Am Mosq Control Assoc*. 1991;7(1):52–5.

Reiter P, Gubler DJ. *Surveillance and Control of Urban Dengue Vectors*. In: Gubler DJ, Kuno G, editors (London, United Kingdom: CAB International, 1997), pp. 425–62.

Reiter P, Lathrop S, Bunning M, Biggerstaff B, Singer D, Tiwari T, Baber L, Amador M, Thirion J, Hayes J, Seca C. Texas lifestyle limits transmission of dengue virus. *Emerg Infect Dis*. 2003;9(1):86–9, https://doi.org/10.3201/eid0901.020220

Reuben R, Das PK, Samuel GD, Brooks GD. Estimation of daily emergence of *Aedes aegypti* (Diptera: Culicidae) in Sonepat, India. *J Med Entomol*. 1978;14:705–14, https://doi.org/10.1093/jmedent/14.6.705

Revay E, Mueller G, Qualls W, Kline D, Naranjo D, Müller G, et al. Control of *Aedes albopictus* with attractive toxic sugar baits (ATSB) and potential impact on non-target organisms in St. Augustine, Florida. *Parasit Res*. 2014;113(1):73–9, https://doi.org/10.1007/s00436-013-3628-4

Rey JR, Nishimura N, Wagner B, Braks MA, O'Connell SM, Lounibos LP. Habitat segregation of mosquito arbovirus vectors in South Florida. *J Med Entomol*. 2006;43(6):1134–41, https://doi.org/10.1603/0022-2585(2006)43[1134:hsomav]2.0.co;2

Richards SL, Ponnusamy L, Unnasch TR, Hassan HK, Apperson CS. Host-feeding patterns of *Aedes albopictus* (Diptera: Culicidae) in relation to availability of human and domestic animals in suburban landscapes of central North Carolina. *J Med Entomol.* 2006;43(3):543–51, https://doi.org/10.1603/0022-2585(2006)43[543:hpoaad]2.0.co;2

Rigau-Pérez JG, Ayala-López A, García-Rivera EJ, Hudson SM, Vorndam V, Reiter P, Cano MP, Clark GG. The reappearance of dengue-3 and a subsequent dengue-4 and dengue-1 epidemic in Puerto Rico in 1998. *Am J Trop Med Hyg.* 2002;67(4):355–62, https://doi.org/10.4269/ajtmh.2002.67.355

Rigau-Perez JG, Gubler DJ. Surveillance for dengue and dengue hemorrhagic fever. In: Gubler DJ, Kuno G, editors. *Dengue and Dengue Hemorrhagic Fever,* (New York, NY: CAB International, 1997, pp. 405–23).

Rigau-Perez JG, Gubler DJ, Vorndam AV, Clark GG. Dengue surveillance--United States, 1986-1992. *MMWR CDC Surveill Summ.* 1994;43(2):7–19.

Rigau-Perez JG, Vorndam AV, Clark GG. The dengue and dengue hemorrhagic fever epidemic in Puerto Rico,1994-1995. *Am J Trop Med Hyg.* 2001 Jan–Feb;64(1–2):67–74, https://doi.org/10.4269/ajtmh.2001.64.67

Ritchie SA. Evolution of dengue control strategies in North Queensland, Australia. *Arbovirus Res Aust.* 2005;9:324–30.

Ritchie SA, Hanna JN, Hills SL, Piispanen JP, McBride WJH, Pyke A, et al. Dengue control in North Queensland, Australia: case recognition and selective indoor residual spraying. *Dengue Bull.* 2002;26:7–13.

Ritchie SA, Long S, Hart A, Webb CE, Russell RC. An adulticidal sticky ovitrap for sampling container-breeding mosquitoes. *J Am Mosq Control Assoc.* 2003;19(3):235–42.

Ritchie SA, Long S, Smith G, Pyke A, Knox TB. Entomological investigations in a focus of dengue transmission in Cairns, Queensland, Australia, by using the sticky ovitraps. *J Med Entomol.* 2004;41(1):1–4, https://doi.org/10.1603/0022-2585-41.1.1

Rodríguez MM, Bisset JA, Fernández D. Levels of insecticide resistance and resistance mechanisms in *Aedes aegypti* from some Latin American countries. *J Am Mosq Control Assoc.* 2007;23(4):420–9, https://doi.org/10.2987/5588.1

Romero-Vivas CM, Wheeler JG, Falconar AK, Romero-Vivas CME, Wheeler JG, Falconar AKI. An inexpensive intervention for the control of larval *Aedes aegypti* assessed by an improved method of surveillance and analysis. *J Am Mosq Control Assoc.* 2002;18(1):40–6.

Ropelewski CF, Halpert MS. Global and regional scale precipitation patterns associated with El Nino / Southern Oscillation. *Mon Weather Rev.* 1987;115:1606–26, https://doi.org/10.1175/1520-0493(1987)115<1606:GARSPP>2.0.CO;2

Rosen L, Rozeboom LE, Sweet BH, Sabin AB. The transmission of dengue by *Aedes polynesiensis* Marks. *Am J Trop Med Hyg*. 1954;3(5):878–82, https://doi.org/10.4269/ajtmh.1954.3.878

Rosenberg R, Lindsey NP, Fischer M, Gregory CJ, Hinckley AF, Mead PS, et al. Vital signs: trends in reported vector-borne disease cases - United States and territories, 2004-2016. *MMWR Morb Mortal Wkly Rep*. 2018;67(17):496–501, https://doi.org/10.15585/mmwr.mm6717e1

Rowe D, McDermott C, Veliz Y, Kerr A, Whiteside M, Coss M, et al. Dengue outbreak response during COVID-19 pandemic, Key Largo, Florida, USA, 2020. *Emerg Infect Dis*. 2023;29(8):1643–7, https://doi.org/10.3201/eid2908.221856

Rueda LM. Pictorial keys for the identification of mosquitoes (Diptera: Culicidae) associated with dengue virus transmission. *Zootaxa*. 2004;589(1):1–60, https://doi.org/10.11646/zootaxa.589.1.1

Russell BM, Kay BH. Calibrated funnel trap for quantifying mosquito (Diptera: Culicidae) abundance in wells. *J Med Entomol*. 1999;36(6):851–5, https://doi.org/10.1093/jmedent/36.6.851

Russell BM, McBride WJH, Mullner H, Kay BH. Epidemiological Significance of subterranean *Aedes aegypti* (Diptera: Culicidae) breeding sites to dengue virus infection in Charters Towers, 1993. *J Med Entomol*. 2002;39(1):143–5, https://doi.org/10.1603/0022-2585-39.1.143

Saleh MS, Abuzinadah OA, Al Ghamdi K, Alsagaf AA, Mahyoub JA. Effectiveness of slow-release tablet formulations of the IGR diflubenzuron and the bioinsecticide spinosad against larvae of *Aedes aegypti* (L.). *African Entomol*. 2013;21(2):349–53.

Salgado V. Studies on the mode of action of spinosad: insect symptoms and physiological correlates. *Pestic Biochem Physiol*. 1998;60(2):91–102, https://doi.org/10.1006/pest.1998.2332

Santiago GA, Vazquez J, Courtney S, Matias KY, Andersen LE, Colon C, et al. Performance of the Trioplex real-time RT-PCR assay for detection of Zika, dengue, and chikungunya viruses. *Nat Commun*. 2018;9(1):1391, https://doi.org/10.1038/s41467-018-03772-1.

Santiago GA, Vergne E, Quiles Y, Cosme J, Vazquez J, Medina JF, et al. Analytical and clinical performance of the CDC real time RT-PCR assay for detection and typing of dengue virus. *PLoS Negl Trop Dis*. 2013;7(7):e2311, https://doi.org/10.1371/journal.pntd.0002311

Savage HM, Niebylski ML, Smith GC, Mitchell CJ, Craig Jr GB. Host-feeding patterns of *Aedes albopictus* (Diptera: Culicidae) at a temperate North American site. *J Med Entomol*. 1993;30(1):27–34, https://doi.org/10.1093/jmedent/30.1.27

Schaffner F, Bellini R, Petrić D, Scholte EJ, Zeller H, Rakotoarivony LM. Development of guidelines for the surveillance of invasive mosquitoes in Europe. *Parasit Vectors*. 2013;6:209, https://doi.org/10.1186/1756-3305-6-209

Schmaedick MA, Ball TS, Burkot TR, Gurr NE. Evaluation of three traps for sampling *Aedes* polynesiensis and other mosquito species in American Samoa. *J Am Mosq Control Assoc*. 2008;24(2):319–22, https://doi.org/10.2987/5652.1

Schneider J, Droll D. *A Timeline for Dengue in the Americas to December 31, 2000 and Noted First Occurrences* (Washington, DC: PAHO, 2001).

Scholte EJ, Takken W, Knols BG. Infection of adult *Aedes aegypti* and *Ae. albopictus* mosquitoes with the entomopathogenic fungus *Metarhizium anisopliae*. *Acta Trop*. 2007;102(3):151–8, https://doi.org/10.1016/j.actatropica.2007.04.011

Scott TW, Clark GG, Lorenz LH, Amerasinghe PH, Reiter P, Edman JD. Detection of multiple blood feeding in *Aedes aegypti* (Diptera: Culicidae) during a single gonotrophic cycle using a histologic technique. *J Med Entomol*. 1993;30(1):94–9, https://doi.org/10.1093/jmedent/30.1.94

Sebastian A, Sein M, Thu M, Corbet P. Suppression of *Aedes aegypti* using augmentative release of dragonfly larvae with community participation in Yangon, Myanmar. *Bull Entomol Res*. 1990;80:223–32.

Sharp TM, Hunsperger E, Santiago GA, Munoz-Jordan JL, Santiago LM, Rivera A, et al. Virus-specific differences in rates of disease during the 2010 dengue epidemic in Puerto Rico. *PLoS Negl Trop Dis*. 2013;7(4):e2159, https://doi.org/10.1371/journal.pntd.0002159

Sharp TM, Lorenzi O, Torres-Velásquez B, Acevedo V, Pérez-Padilla J, Rivera A, et al. Autocidal gravid ovitraps protect humans from chikungunya virus infection by reducing *Aedes aegypti* mosquito populations. *PLoS Negl Trop Dis*. 2019;13(7):e0007538, https://doi.org/10.1371/journal.pntd.0007538

Sharp TM, Tufa AJ, Cotter CJ, Lozier MJ, Santiago GA, Johnson SS, et al. Identification of risk factors and mosquito vectors associated with dengue virus infection in American Samoa, 2017. *Plos Glob Public Health*. 2023;3(7):e0001604, https://doi.org/10.1371/journal.pgph.0001604

Sheppard PM, Macdonald WW, Tonn RJ. A new method of measuring the relative prevalence of *Aedes aegypti*. *Bull WHO*. 1969;40(3):467–8.

Shope R. Global climate change and infectious diseases. *Environ Health Perspect*. 1991;96:171–4, https://doi.org/10.1289/ehp.9196171

Sippy R, Rivera GE, Sanchez V, Heras F, Morejón B, Beltrán E, et al. Ingested insecticide to control *Aedes aegypti*: developing a novel dried attractive toxic sugar bait device for intra-domiciliary control. *Parasit Vectors*. 2020;13(1):78, https://doi.org/10.1186/s13071-020-3930-9

Siqueira-Junior JB, Maciel IJ, Barcellos C, Souza WV, Carvalho MS, Nascimento NE, et al. Spatial point analysis based on dengue surveys at household level in central Brazil. *BMC Public Health*. 2008;8:361, https://doi.org/10.1186/1471-2458-8-361

Sissoko F, Junnila A, Traore MM, Traore SF, Doumbia S, Dembele SM, et al. Frequent sugar feeding behavior by *Aedes aegypti* in Bamako, Mali makes them ideal candidates for control with attractive toxic sugar baits (ATSB). *PLoS One*. 2019;14(6):e0214170, https://doi.org/10.1371/journal.pone.0214170

Soper FL. *Aedes aegypti* and yellow fever. *Bull World Health Organ*. 1967;36(4):521–7.

Stoddard PK. Managing *Aedes aegypti* populations in the first Zika transmission zones in the continental United States. *Acta Trop*. 2018;187:108–18, https://doi.org/10.1016/j.actatropica.2018.07.031

Strickman D. Longevity of *Aedes aegypti* (Diptera: Culicidae) compared in cages and field under ambient conditions in rural Thailand. *Southeast Asian J Trop Med Public Health*. 2006;37(3):456–62.

Strickman D. Area repellent products. In: Debboun M, Frances SP, Strickman D, editors. *Insect Repellents: Principles, Methods, and Uses*, (Boca Raton, FL: CRC Press, 2007, pp. 385–93).

Sutherland GL, Nasci RS. Detection of West Nile virus in large pools of mosquitoes. *J Am Mosq Control Assoc*. 2007;23(4):389–95, https://doi.org/10.2987/5630.1

Tambwe MM, Moore SJ, Chilumba H, Swai JK, Moore JD, Stica C, et al. Semi-field evaluation of freestanding transfluthrin passive emanators and the BG sentinel trap as a "push-pull control strategy" against *Aedes aegypti* mosquitoes. *Parasit Vectors*. 2020;13(1):392, https://doi.org/10.1186/s13071-020-04263-3

Tambwe MM, Saddler A, Kibondo UA, Mashauri R, Kreppel KS, Govella NJ, et al. Semi-field evaluation of the exposure-free mosquito electrocuting trap and BG-Sentinel trap as an alternative to the human landing catch for measuring the efficacy of transfluthrin emanators against *Aedes aegypti*. *Parasit Vectors*. 2021;14(1):265, https://doi.org/10.1186/s13071-021-04754-x

Tan CH, Wong PS, Li MZ, Vythilingam I, Ng LC. Evaluation of the dengue NS1 Ag Strip(R) for detection of dengue virus antigen in *Aedes aegypti* (Diptera: Culicidae). *Vector Borne Zoonotic Dis*. 2011;11(6):789–92, https://doi.org/10.1089/vbz.2010.0028

Teixeira MD, Barreto ML, Costa MDN, Ferreira LDA, Vasconcelos PFC, Cairncross S. Dynamics of dengue virus circulation: a silent epidemic in a complex urban area. *Trop Med Int Health*. 2002;7(9):757–62, https://doi.org/10.1046/j.1365-3156.2002.00930.x

Trout RT, Brown GC, Potter MF, Hubbard JL. Efficacy of two pyrethroid insecticides applied as barrier treatments for managing mosquito (Diptera: Culicidae) populations in suburban residential properties. *J Med Entomol.* 2007;44(3):470–7, https://doi.org/10.1603/0022-2585(2007)44[470:eotpia]2.0.co;2

Trpis M, Hausermann W. Dispersal and other population parameters of *Aedes aegypti* in an African village and their possible significance in epidemiology of vector-borne diseases. *Am J Trop Med Hyg.* 1986;35:1263–79, https://doi.org/10.4269/ajtmh.1986.35.1263

Tun-Lin W, Kay BH, Barnes A, Tun-Lin W, Kay BH, Barnes A. Understanding productivity, a key to *Aedes aegypti* surveillance. *Am J Trop Med Hyg.* 1995;53(6):595–601, https://doi.org/10.4269/ajtmh.1995.53.595

Unlu I, Rochlin I, Suman DS, Wang Y, Chandel K, Gaugler R. Large-scale operational pyriproxyfen autodissemination deployment to suppress the immature Asian tiger mosquito (Diptera: Culicidae) populations. *J Med Entomol.* 2020;57(4):1120–30, https://doi.org/10.1093/jme/tjaa011

Urdaneta L, Herrera F, Pernalete M, Zoghbi N, Rubio-Palis Y, Barrios R, et al. Detection of dengue viruses in field-caught *Aedes aegypti* (Diptera: Culicidae) in Maracay, Aragua state, Venezuela by type-specific polymerase chain reaction. *Infect Gen Evol.* 2005;5(2):177–84, https://doi.org/10.1016/j.meegid.2004.09.004

Utarini A, Indriani C, Ahmad RA, Tantowijoyo W, Arguni E, Ansari MR, et al. Efficacy of *Wolbachia*-infected mosquito deployments for the control of dengue. *N Engl J Med.* 2021;384(23):2177–86, https://doi.org/10.1056/NEJMoa2030243

Valerio L, Marini F, Bongiorno G, Facchinelli L, Pombi M, Caputo B, Maroli M, Della Torre A. Host-feeding patterns of *Aedes albopictus* (Diptera: Culicidae) in urban and rural contexts within Rome Province, Italy. *Vector Borne Zoonotic Dis.* 2010;10:291–4, https://doi.org/10.1089/vbz.2009.0007

Van Kleef E, Bambrick HJ, Hales S. The geographic distribution of dengue fever and the potential influence of global climate change. *TropIKA. net.* 2010, https://journal.tropika.net/scielo.php?script=sci_arttext&pid=S2078-86062010005000001

Vanlerberghe V, Villegas E, Oviedo M, Baly A, Lenhart A, McCall PJ, et al. Evaluation of the effectiveness of insecticide treated materials for household level dengue vector control. *PLoS Negl Trop Dis.* 2011;5(3):e994, https://doi.org/10.1371/journal.pntd.0000994

Vanlerberghe V, Gómez-Dantés H, Vazquez-Prokopec G, Alexander N, Manrique-Saide P, Coelho G, et al. Changing paradigms in *Aedes* control: considering the spatial heterogeneity of dengue transmission. *Rev Panam Salud Publica.* 2017;41:e16.

Vasilakis N, Cardosa J, Hanley KA, Holmes EC, Weaver SC. Fever from the forest: prospects for the continued emergence of sylvatic dengue virus and its impact on public health. *Nat Rev Microbiol.* 2011;9:532–41, https://doi.org/10.1038/nrmicro2595

Vazquez-Prokopec GM, Galvin WA, Kelly R, Kitron U. A new, cost-effective, battery-powered aspirator for adult mosquito collections. *J Med Entomol.* 2009;46(6):1256–9, https://doi.org/10.1603/033.046.0602

Vazquez-Prokopec GM, Kitron U, Montgomery B, Horne P, Ritchie SA. Quantifying the spatial dimension of dengue virus epidemic spread within a tropical urban environment. *PLoS Negl Trop Dis.* 2010;21;4(12):e920, https://doi.org/10.1371/journal.pntd.0000920

Voge NV, Sanchez-Vargas I, Blair CD, Eisen L, Beaty BJ. Detection of dengue virus NS1 antigen in infected *Aedes aegypti* using a commercially available kit. *Am J Trop Med Hyg.* 2013;88(2):260–6, https://doi.org/10.4269/ajtmh.2012.12-0477

Wang Y, An M, Stevens KM, Liu N. Insecticide resistance in Alabama populations of the mosquito *Aedes albopictus. J Med Entomol.* 2022;59(5):1678–86, https://doi.org/10.1093/jme/tjac085

Washburn JO, Hartmann EU. Could *Aedes albopictus* (Diptera, Culicidae) become established in California tree holes? *J Med Entomol.* 1992;29(6):995–1005, https://doi.org/10.1093/jmedent/29.6.995

Waterman SH, Novak RJ, Sather GE, Bailey RE, Rios I, Gubler DJ. Dengue transmission in two Puerto Rican communities in 1982. *Am J Trop Med Hyg.* 1985;34(3):625–32, https://doi.org/10.4269/ajtmh.1985.34.625

Watts AG, Miniota J, Joseph HA, Brady OJ, Kraemer MU, Grills AW, Morrison S, Esposito DH, Nicolucci A, German M, Creatore MI. Elevation as a proxy for mosquito-borne Zika virus transmission in the Americas. *PLoS One.* 2017;12(5):e0178211, https://doi.org/10.1371/journal.pone.0178211

Watts DM, Burke DS, Harrison BA, Whitmire RE, Nisalak A. Effect of temperature on the vector efficiency of *Aedes aegypti* for dengue-2 virus. *Am J Trop Med Hyg.* 1987;36(1):143–52.

Wilke ABB, Vasquez C, Mauriello PJ, Beier JC. Ornamental bromeliads of Miami-Dade County, Florida are important breeding sites for *Aedes aegypti* (Diptera: Culicidae). *Parasit Vectors.* 2018;11(1):283, https://doi.org/10.1186/s13071-018-2866-9

Williams CR, Long SA, Russell RC, Ritchie SA. Field efficacy of the BG-Sentinel compared with CDC Backpack Aspirators and CO2-baited EVS traps for collection of adult *Aedes aegypti* in Cairns, Queensland, Australia. *J Am Mosq Control Assoc.* 2006;22(2):296–300, https://doi.org/10.2987/8756-971X(2006)22[296:FEOTBC]2.0.CO;2

Williams CR, Long SA, Webb CE, Bitzhenner M, Geier M, Russell RC, et al. *Aedes aegypti* population sampling using BG-Sentinel traps in North

Queensland Australia: statistical considerations for trap deployment and sampling strategy. *J Med Entomol*. 2007;44(2):345–50, https://doi.org/10.1603/0022-2585(2007)44[345:aapsub]2.0.co;2

Wilton DP, Kloter KO. Preliminary evaluation of a black cylinder suction trap for *Aedes aegypti* and *Culex quinquefasciatus* (Diptera: Culicidae). *J Med Entomol*. 1985;22(1):113–4, https://doi.org/10.1093/jmedent/22.1.113

Wise de Valdez MR, Nimmo D, Betz J, Gong HF, James AA, Alphey L, et al. Genetic elimination of dengue vector mosquitoes. *Proc Natl Acad Sci U S A*. 2011;108(12):4772–5, https://doi.org/10.1073/pnas.1019295108

Withanage GP, Viswakula SD, Gunawardene YS, Hapugoda MD. Use of Novaluron-based Autocidal Gravid Ovitraps to control *Aedes* dengue vector mosquitoes in the District of Gampaha, Sri Lanka. *Biomed Res Int*. 2020;2020:9567019, https://doi.org/10.1155/2020/9567019

WHO. *Dengue: Guidelines for Diagnosis, Treatment, Prevention and Control: New Edition*, World Health Organization. (Geneva, Switzerland: WHO, 2009, p. 147).

WHO. *Monitoring and Managing Insecticide Resistance in Aedes Mosquito Populations*, (Geneva, Switzerland: WHO, 2016).

WHO. *Efficacy-Testing of Traps for Control of Aedes spp. Mosquito Vectors* (Geneva: WHO, 2018). [cited 19 May 2025]. Available from: https://eprints.gla.ac.uk/173660/1/173660.pdf

WHO. Global dengue surveillance [Internet]. World Health Organization;2025 [cited 19 May 2025]. Available from: https://worldhealthorg.shinyapps.io/dengue_global/

Wu HH, Wang CY, Teng HJ, Lin C, Lu LC, Jian SW, et al. A dengue vector surveillance by human population-stratified ovitrap survey for *Aedes* (Diptera: Culicidae) adult and egg collections in high dengue-risk areas of Taiwan. *J Med Entomol*. 2013;50(2):261–9, https://doi.org/10.1603/me11263

Xue R, Ali A, Day JF. Commercially available insect repellents and criteria for their use. In: Debboun M, Frances SP, Strickman D, editors. *Insect Repellents: Principles, Methods, and Uses* (Boca Raton, FL: CRC Press, 2007, pp. 405–15).

Xue RD, Ali A, Kline DL, Barnard DR. Field evaluation of boric acid- and fipronil-based bait stations against adult mosquitoes. *J Am Mosq Control Assoc*. 2008;24(3):415–8, https://doi.org/10.2987/5683.1

Zeller H, Van Bortel W, Sudre B. Chikungunya: Its history in Africa and Asia and its spread to new regions in 2013-2014. *J Infect Dis*. 2016;214(suppl 5):S436–40, https://doi.org/10.1093/infdis/jiw391

Zhong D, Lo E, Hu R, Metzger ME, Cummings R, Bonizzoni M, et al. Genetic analysis of invasive *Aedes albopictus* populations in Los Angeles County, California and its potential public health impact. *PLoS One*. 2013;8(7):e68586, https://doi.org/10.1371/journal.pone.0068586

Index

About the Team

Alessandra Tosi was the managing editor for this book.

Annie Hine proof-read this manuscript and compiled the index.

Jeevanjot Kaur Nagpal designed the cover. The cover was produced in InDesign using the Fontin font.

Annie typeset the book in InDesign and produced the paperback and hardback editions. The main text font is Tex Gyre Pagella and the heading font is Californian FB.

Jeremy Bowman produced the EPUB and PDF editions.

The conversion to the HTML edition was performed with epublius, an open-source software which is freely available on our GitHub page at https://github.com/OpenBookPublishers

Hannah Shakespeare was in charge of marketing.

This book was peer-reviewed by two anonymous referees. Experts in their field, these readers give their time freely to help ensure the academic rigour of our books. We are grateful for their generous and invaluable contributions.

This book need not end here...

Share

All our books — including the one you have just read — are free to access online so that students, researchers and members of the public who can't afford a printed edition will have access to the same ideas. This title will be accessed online by hundreds of readers each month across the globe: why not share the link so that someone you know is one of them?

This book and additional content is available at
https://doi.org/10.11647/OBP.0472

Donate

Open Book Publishers is an award-winning, scholar-led, not-for-profit press making knowledge freely available one book at a time. We don't charge authors to publish with us: instead, our work is supported by our library members and by donations from people who believe that research shouldn't be locked behind paywalls.

Join the effort to free knowledge by supporting us at
https://www.openbookpublishers.com/support-us

You may also be interested in:

Intellectual Property and Public Health in the Developing World

Monirul Azam

https://doi.org/10.11647/OBP.0093

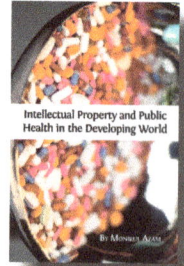

The Economics of Cultural Loss

Harm and Resilience in North American Indigenous Communities

Mukesh Eswaran

https://doi.org/10.11647/OBP.0477

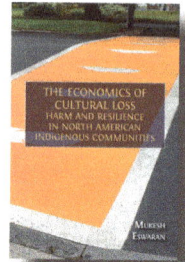

Non-communicable Disease Prevention

Best Buys, Wasted Buys and Contestable Buys

Edited by Wanrudee Isaranuwatchai, Rachel A. Archer, Yot Teerawattananon, and Anthony J. Culyer

https://doi.org/10.11647/OBP.0195

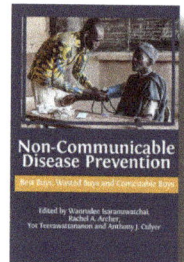

A Complete Guide to Maggot Therapy

Clinical Practice, Therapeutic Principles, Production, Distribution, and Ethics

Edited by Frank Stadler

https://doi.org/10.11647/obp.0300

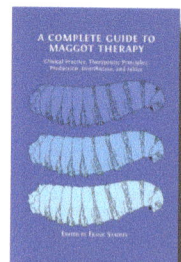

www.ingramcontent.com/pod-product-compliance
Lightning Source LLC
Chambersburg PA
CBHW041145230326
41599CB00039BA/7183